I'm Champion
Call Me Bob

Bob Champion
MBE

FCM Publishing
Lincoln, UK

Dedication

To Janette, Mary, Lillian & all my family.

To my friends & fellow jockeys
Lucy, Howard, Derek, Jonathan, Jim and Ian,

and also to
Josh and Nick for without their loyalty there
wouldn't be a story.

Acknowledgements

First and foremost, to my family and friends, thanks as ever for all of your support. I may not say it often, but you are my life.

Thanks also to Mike Cattermole for writing the foreword to this book. Your kind words are very humbling.

I also want to thank all of you who have supported me and the Bob Champion Cancer Trust throughout the years. From the smallest of individual donations to the biggest of corporate assistance, the money, time and effort you have given have been critical in our success.

It is very important for me to put on record that the achievements of the Trust, which bears my name, are wholly down to the dedication, professionalism and innovation of the scientists, researchers, doctors and nurses who have given of their skills and expertise. The advances they have enabled are quite staggering and a fitting testament to their abilities.

Finally, I'd personally like to thank Taryn Johnston and Ian Hooper for all their support and encouragement in the production of this, my updated biography. I couldn't have done it without them.

Table of Contents

Foreword

When Bob Champion won the 1981 Grand National on Aldaniti, I was in my second year as a student at Keele University.

I had actually had a bet on Spartan Missile and 54-year-old John Thorne, who came home in second place. I remember feeling a little sorry for Mr Thorne but those sentiments were soon overwhelmed by the realisation that I was watching an incredible sporting story unfolding before my eyes.

Let's face it, if you had written a script about a man who had been diagnosed with cancer and given weeks to live only to recover and return to ride in and then win the world's scariest and most charismatic horse race - and on a horse who had also looked to be at the end of the road - they would have smiled at you and shown you the door.

Even now, decades on, I truly believe that Bob's is the greatest sporting story ever told, an unrivalled personal triumph gained over the worst of adversities.

I also always felt that Bob's tale was an even better one because he was a Champion by name, too. Perfect.

His story will be familiar to many of you but not to some younger readers perhaps, which is why Bob and Taryn Johnston felt it needed a revisit. And, things have moved on too, of course.

You may wonder if the rest of Bob's life has been an anti-climax since that sunniest of days at Aintree. However, nothing could be further from the truth because his starting the Bob Champion Cancer Trust with Nick and Valda Embiricos, Aldaniti's owners, has meant that he has more than embellished and sustained his legacy.

The Trust's work continues apace and to date it has raised more than £12m for research into male urological cancers. I know he is extremely proud of that and now, he even has a huge modern scientific building named after him at the Norwich Research Park.

There's enough there to think that Bob would have long been carried away by his own ego but to meet him is to meet one of the world's good people. His is such an easy, gentle presence, totally unpretentious, thoroughly genuine and he is amusing too, sometimes unwittingly.

Every other year we have a carol concert for the Trust. It's a posh do, held at the wonderful and historic Chelsea Old Church and attended by some of west London's finest.

Bob has to do a reading and gets quite nervous about it. The line "gold, frankincense and myrrh" was causing him to be anxious and he turned to me and said: "I know I am going to muck this up, I will probably say Frankenstein instead."

Well, talk about talking yourself into it! Bob duly delivered the line, which included the title of Mary Shelley's famous book, and I doubt whether any congregation over the centuries at Chelsea Old Church sniggered like they did that evening – in the most sympathetic way of course.

It was typical of Bob that he laughed along with us. It didn't matter. He, of all people, will know that there are plenty more important things out there that do indeed need to be taken seriously, and finding a cure for cancer is most certainly one of them.

Enjoy the book.

Mike Cattermole

"For the life of me I don't know why he's not Sir Bob Champion. Of all the people, footballers, pop stars and the like that receive Knighthoods, to me Bob deserves it for everything he's done."
Derek Thompson

The Almost
Impossible Jump

It's not every day you get told you're going to die.

I was a thirty-one-year old professional jockey. A National Hunt jump jockey to be precise. In sporting circles, we're considered to be amongst the fittest and strongest, pound for pound, of any sportsmen or women. So I was very physically fit. I had my own car, my own house and my own hair. I was even known to have had quite some success with the ladies. To be told I'd be dead within the year, probably inside four to five months, had left me shell-shocked. I was numb. The doctor's words drifted over me, around me, without really registering. Then, as I properly focused on what was being said, I felt a new feeling. Terror.

"You have testicular cancer, Bob. It's confirmed and it's spread to your chest."

I looked at my reflection in the room's long mirror. I looked remarkably healthy, all things considered.

The doctor continued to talk. She was being professionally dispassionate. I imagine it's how you need to be when dealing with life and death, when you're telling the worst news to patients. Trying to explain how bad things were. I mean, I knew things weren't great. After all, I'd already been subjected to two exploratory operations, the first of which had removed one of my testicles, but I had convinced myself that it was all going to be a non-event. Honestly, I had. I'd thought about the prospect of it being cancer and soundly dismissed it. It couldn't be. I wouldn't let it be.

"…but the treatment is so much more effective nowadays… although it's invasive…"

I thought it was just some random lump. No way was it cancer. Cancer? I couldn't get cancer. Old people, smokers, heavy drinkers, all of which I wasn't, they got cancer. I rode horses for goodness sake. I was an outdoors type. Fit, healthy, young. I couldn't have cancer.

"…it will mean you have to stop riding…"

Those words made it through to me. I couldn't stop riding.

My 'job' had both thrilled and inspired me for over ten years. It was all I had. It couldn't be coming to an end. Anyway, I figured being a National Hunt jump jockey was always risky. It's one of the few sports where an ambulance follows the competitors in real-time. I knew all those risks. Lived them. Suffered most of them. The falls, the breaks, the concussions. It was all part of the game. I knew my way around hospital wards and how to discharge myself early with broken fingers and ankles and ribs. Waking up the following morning after a heavy fall, unable to move any part of my body without agony, but this… No this wasn't anything I knew about. Don't get me wrong, I knew they weren't telling me lies. I knew there had been a problem with my testicle and I'd been urged to have it checked out. I just never expected this.

In my mind I thought the most dangerous thing I faced came with four legs and hurtled towards big fences. A cancer ward and chemotherapy wasn't an end I could have imagined.

The woman doctor, Jane, finished speaking. I realised I hadn't heard most of what she had said. Her male companion started talking. I tried again to focus on what I was being told.

"…radical new treatment…"

Then I realised both of them were looking at me. Waiting for me to say something. I tried to think of a reasonable question, other than screaming 'No!' at the top of my lungs. My mind whirled with the little I knew about cancer treatments. I eventually managed, "Can I have radiation?"

"I'm afraid, your cancer is already at stage three. Radiation treatment won't do for it. If this was even a decade ago, nothing would do for it. But, Bob, there is a new treatment that's been pioneered in America. A new type of chemotherapy."

"So I will be able to keep riding?"

The question threw him off. "Ummm, for a few months, perhaps," he said, and looked a little puzzled.

Looking back it seems surreal that all I was concerned about was riding. But it's the truth. It was my life and I'd just had my most successful season to date. If I couldn't ride, they could stuff their treatment.

"National Hunt riding is dangerous, Doc. Jockeys get hurt and some die. I'd rather take my chances on the back of a horse than curling up in a hospital bed," I said, with as much bravado as I could manage.

I know now that the two doctors hadn't ever had a patient say no before. Most patients grasped on to the chance of life with both hands, so for this plain-spoken Yorkshire man to sit in front of them and say, "No thanks," was a bit of a mystery to them.

Jane said, "That's daft, Bob. You could live for a few months at most or, you could take this new treatment and have the rest of your life ahead of you. It's silly if you don't take the treatment."

"But I'll have to stop riding eventually if I have this?" I asked, still not focussing on the very real prospect of dying.

"Well yes. Perhaps for a year, perhaps for good," she said.

I felt angry. They just weren't getting it. I was a top jump jockey to one of the top trainers in the country. I couldn't just 'not ride'. It didn't work like that. I'd never come back from that type of 'career break'. No trainer would ring me up if they thought I was ill and certainly they wouldn't be ringing me up after months out of the saddle.

The argument went back and forth. I can still see the surprise on their faces as I said, "No thanks," again and again. Thank goodness they were as stubborn as me.

They insisted on telling me what was ahead of me and how the chemotherapy was producing marvellous results. I continued to say no. I wasn't thinking about the cancer. I was thinking about my career. Or perhaps, and it has taken me a lot of years to reconcile this, perhaps, I had already given up and chosen just to die.

No grand gestures you understand, I just knew about riding, it was how I lived my life. Perhaps I thought I could go out in a more fitting way? Maybe a bad fall would end things like they were supposed to? What did I know of chemotherapy? I was just a jockey.

I told them that there was no way I was wasting away in a hospital bed having people fuss over me, that's not who I was. I told the doctors straight out that I'd take my chances without the treatment.

Jane stood up and told me to listen to her as she explained what the treatment actually did. How I would need at least four cycles of it, each one lasting 21-days. She told me what this new drug, developed in the USA, could do for me. She explained that I'd be violently sick, lose my hair and suffer agonising constipation, as well as succumbing to anorexia. Her sales pitch definitely needed work. None of what she told me sounded like a great idea. It certainly didn't sell the treatment as far as I was concerned!

Then came the real kicker. Almost undoubtedly, I would be sterile. Unable to have children. I had never realised how important that was to me. It somehow made me feel… less. Less than a man.

Back and forth and me still ignoring them, and then I'm not sure where the question came from, but I remember asking, "Okay, bottom line, what are my chances? Exactly?"

Perhaps it was a moment of inspiration on the doctors' part, but they swapped the language of medicine for a language I understood. Jane spoke of the odds of a recovery. She related it to my everyday life. She said, if I started the treatment immediately, I'd have a thirty five to forty percent chance of a full recovery.

Her colleague piped in, "Look Bob, with no treatment, you're dead in five months. With treatment you have a chance. A good chance. What would you say if I gave you a 6-to-4 option in a novice chase, would you ride it?"

I'm just a jockey, but I understand odds. A 6-4 in a novice chase was doable. I'd have a wager on that. I'd definitely have taken the ride. It seemed reasonable. Yet it was so hard to square the starkness of the whole situation, when I felt as well as I did. I think that was why I couldn't come to terms with the real circumstances of what I was facing. The spectre of my death wasn't making me feel ill, wasn't tearing at my body, wasn't destroying me from the inside out. Well, not yet.

I couldn't process the finality of what I was actually dealing with and other things flitted through my head. Daft nonsense looking back, but then they seemed important. Things like; I really hated the thought of going bald. I know, it may seem stupid given that my life was at risk, but the tanned fit man looking at me from the mirror couldn't see the illness inside that was killing him.

The final doubt and the one most crucial to me, was whether I'd ride again following the treatment. It was going to be invasive, with massive side effects. Both doctors didn't think I'd ride again, especially due to the expected lung damage that would be caused by the chemotherapy, but they once again gave me the odds. They once again gave me hope and said it would depend on how I responded to the treatment. I know now that both of them didn't think there was a cat in hell's chance of me making it back into the saddle, but they didn't say that. Thank goodness. It wouldn't have been the 'done thing' to tell this nut of a patient that he really was nuts.

It was Monday the 13th August 1979 and I recall with the clarity of it being yesterday, that I said to myself if I was going to do this I needed to set a goal. One that would prove them all wrong. The only one that mattered to me, the only one that made sense. I was going to get better, come back and win the Grand National on a horse called Aldaniti. It was that clear in my head. I repeated it to myself.

So, against everything I felt inside, but with that crystal clear goal in mind, I agreed to start the treatment. It would begin that evening. Had I known what I had just let myself in for, I wouldn't have gone ahead.

Given all that my life was to become, I'm glad I did.

Under Starter's Orders

A bed of stinging nettles.

That's what I fell into the very first time I jumped a pony over an obstacle. I was four and it hurt. A lot. The landing was soft and cushioning, so I had no broken bones, but each time I tried to get out, I got stung even more. It left a very lasting impression on a young body and mind. I knew that I was not for jumping anything on a horse again. Ever.

Now, my Dad plonking me on a horse at four and making me jump a fence, regardless of how small it was, might seem a bit strange, but I don't want you thinking he was an unkind man. He wasn't. Just a bit driven. Mind you, he was allowed to be. He'd gone off to the Second World War and come back from Arnhem with a right arm that was severely wounded. It could have been, perhaps should have been, the end of his riding days, but the men who came back from the war were a different breed and my Dad never contemplated giving up. After twelve months in hospital recovering from Leptospirosis, or what they called 'the black jaundice' and with an arm that had a permanent lack of feeling and strength, he returned to riding with the local hunt.

Old Bob, as he was known after my arrival on the scene, was the seventh generation of horseman in our family. In proper terms, he and the rest had been professional huntsmen. Not woodchoppers like some Disney movie, but huntsmen who hunt the hounds, within the traditional horse and hound hunts that were throughout rural England. My Dad started off down in Kent, then moved to Sussex before being offered the post of the Cleveland Pack up in Yorkshire, just after I was born. We moved up there and that's where I grew up. It makes me a Yorkshire man, through and through, but I was actually born in Sussex on the 4th June 1948.

Sussex or Yorkshire, it didn't matter. The move didn't change my heritage. I was going to be the eighth generation of huntsmen and Old Bob was going to make sure of it. He was a magnificent horseman my Dad. Definitely old school in his thoughts and methods, but my goodness could he handle horses. Be it riding them, getting them to jump or training and breaking them. By the time I was four, I had already been trotting around on ponies, but Dad obviously thought it was time for me to learn how to jump. He put a small ladder down on its side. The pony went over and I went sailing off into the soft, yet stingy, landing. I think me falling into the nettles and my subsequent unwillingness to go anywhere near a horse for a while, was a major disappointment for him. But we got over it. With the help of a very pretty girl and her pony. But that comes later.

It's been said over the years that I have 'Champion Charm' and that accounts for my later success with the ladies. I'm not so sure about that. My Dad however, well that's a different story! Women would swoon over him and he always looked as though he'd been poured into his scarlet hunting jacket. I know many a village lady thought he was so handsome and charming, but truth be told he was a hard, disciplining man who perhaps had too much fondness for a drink. However, I know for certain that had he not been so hard on me and had I had a softer father, I'd not be the man I am today. In fact, I'd not be here today as I wouldn't have survived the cancer. He taught me that no matter what was thrown at you, you got up and fought back.

Before we leave my Dad's background, I should say something about hunting. I realise the issue is, of course, controversial, but, having grown up with hunting packs, I have a different viewpoint to some. Certainly different to that so vehemently expressed by many who had never seen a hunt in the run up to the passing of the Hunting Act of 2004. I was back then and still am now, happy to explain my thoughts on it. I am content in thinking how the rural necessity to keep the native fox population in check was well met by the hunt. How the pack and the traditions surrounding it was a mainstay of rural life and not just one enjoyed by some upper-class elite that many would paint it. I could argue how the fox population, undealt with, has become a nuisance and how the over-population has led to the increase in foxes now so prevalent in urban settings. All of which will be of no consequence to those opposed to hunting and for each argument I can come up with, they will counter with their own. It is what it is. I have my opinion, but am fully accepting of the passing of the law in line with the majority's sentiment. I just want to point out that being a huntsman did not make my father, nor the other people involved with the hunt, bad people. They were of their time and were neither cruel nor blood-thirsty.

My Mum, Phyllis was quietly spoken and demur in comparison to my Dad. I'm looking back a long time and society has changed, but she was to me, 'a proper mum'. Always there, at the centre of my world, the strength of the family. The cohesion. Mum may not have spoken loudly, but she controlled my sister, Mary and I and we never knew her to be wrong about anything. She came from good old-fashioned farming stock and how lucky we were to have her. She made all our meals, made and mended our clothes and read to Mary and me at night. I know all children think their mum's cooking was the best, (my Mum's was by the way), but what was definitely certain, regardless of bias, was how good a seamstress she was. My goodness could she sew. She could make the latest designs just from looking at the pattern and in later years she'd be much in demand with local, 'top-end' fashion stores as an alterations tailor. Mary reminded me that when I was about eight, Mum had made me a shirt and I wore it so much it became thread-bare to the point that even Mum's talents couldn't rescue it, so she put it in the bin. I was outraged and promptly took it out and continued to wear it. I always was Mum's favourite, as Mary is keen to tell anyone who'll listen!

Mary is my younger sister by eighteen months. Oh, this is hard to admit, even now, when I am old enough to know better about sibling rivalries, but she was the best rider out of all of us. She excelled at it. By the way, I shall confess that we have shared a feisty and volatile relationship all our lives. I was a horror to her when she was little. I remember one day the school bus picking up our friends and driving away leaving me and Mary fighting in the bottom of a muddy ditch. But she was and always will be my little sister. So she and I were allowed, and are still allowed, to fight. Far be it though, that anyone from outside tries to pick on her. That feeling was and is mutual. I suppose I should recount a time when trailing along behind us, as little sisters do, she saw some bigger boys take our conkers off us and give us a hard time. Well, she flew at them, kicking and shouting until she got our conkers back. You didn't mess with Mary even then! I'd often torment her, as older brothers do, then I'd promise to give her my toys if she didn't tell Mum and Dad. She never told and of course, I never gave her my toys!

So that was the four of us. Living in rural Yorkshire in the late Forties and Fifties, with my father running both the Hunt's kennels and a knackering service. For those who may not know what knackering is, simply put, it's how you dispose of any dead animals that aren't fit for human consumption. A Knacker is a licensed person who takes the carcass away and renders it into those by-products that can be used in other trades. Obviously, there were a lot more working animals back then and wherever they could be found in numbers there was a requirement for a 'Knacker'.

Life in those days was fairly simple and straightforward. It does sound rather like a cliché, but it is true, that we didn't have a lot of money and yes, there was a tin bath filled up in front of the fire and yes, we did take it in turns so as not to waste water. However, because of the hunt we always had horses, although after my bed of nettles, I preferred walking the hounds for exercise.

At age eight, I would often be found helping out on the next door neighbour's farm. It was owned by two brothers, Percy and Herbert and their sister, Miss Seaton. We never knew her first name, but she always made me a Battenberg cake which I still love

9

to this day. Percy encouraged me to start up my own rabbit business and he arranged for me to supply the local butcher. They were very good to me and used to let me keep all the profits. They'd also let me drive the tractor and help with the ploughing. It turns out I was quite good at that and even won a few ploughing competitions, but I didn't care much for cows, especially the milking, something that would follow me into my teenage years on my Uncle's farm. But I loved all the farm machinery and driving tractors. Although, when I rule the world, I'd ban them from being allowed to drive on roads during daylight hours. In fact, if I ever stand for Parliament, that may be a cornerstone of my manifesto. I also loved fishing and on occasion I'd go to work with my Dad on his knackering rounds.

By this stage, I had already met my two best friends, brothers Howard and Derek Thompson. I am so lucky to say we remain just the same to this day. We'd met on the hunt and as their parents were friends with mine, they'd often come to our house and we'd play together. It wasn't long before their house became my second home and Mrs Thompson will forever be my second mother. She has always treated me as one of her boys and is still as bright as a button today at the grand age of 99!

Howard and Derek went to a different school to me, but in the holidays I would go with Mr and Mrs Thompson to pick them up and then, for the rest of the school-break, Howard, Derek and I would go everywhere together. This included Redcar races with my Dad in his knacker's van. He'd park up opposite the winning post and the grandstand, just across from the television commentary box. One day, I guess an interviewee hadn't shown up and the ITV front man, John Rickman, obviously desperate to fill a bit of air time grabbed all three of us boys. He asked us the obvious question, 'What do you want to be when you grow up?' It's a weird and wonderful thing, but because we are all still friends we can remember what we said that day. Howard announced he wanted to be a jockey. I said I wanted to win the Grand National and Derek, or Tommo as he would be called by everyone else in the future, said he wanted to be a race commentator like Peter O'Sullevan. It's a shame that Howard, the best rider out of all of us, never fulfilled his ambition, although he did manage a few point-to-point victories. Instead, he took on his family business and he and his partner Tina Jackson have their own stables. I'm pleased to say he still makes time for the races. We all know what happened to me and as for Tommo, well he did indeed go on to have, and still has, a tremendously successful media career, including being the face of Channel-4 Racing for nearly thirty years.

If you are into racing then you know him as, Tommo, but I've always called him Derek, so that's how I'll refer to him throughout the rest of my book.

It was always a safe bet that with all the horsemen in my family history, I wasn't going to be staying out of a saddle forever. So, at eight or nine I was ready to try again. I just wasn't ready to try in front of onlookers. Instead, I'd saddle up my pony and go off into the countryside alone. Over time my confidence grew and I did get a lot of help from a family friend called Margaret Silman. She encouraged me to go hunting but when I was still hesitant taking on jumps she went to extraordinary lengths to help me. She would ride alongside me until we came to the obstacle, then she'd jump it first, tether her horse, come back, take my pony, jump it over and then wait for me to scramble through to the other side.

I used to work at the hunt kennels and at fourteen, I was a few years older than Bobby and Mary, so I would look after them during the hunt and take them out on the lead.

Bobby was not the bravest of riders and I don't think horses were really his first love. I was always so surprised that he became a jockey as he always said he wanted to be a chef. He loved to cook. I can't remember what his speciality was or if it was even edible, but I know it would often contain bananas!

We would call him 'Little Bob' in deference to his Dad and as time moved on and I got married, I would often say to my husband that I'd spoken to 'Little Bob'. On returning home one day my husband found a handsome young man sunbathing in the garden, he demanded to know who it was and when I said 'Little Bob' he replied shortly,

"Well he's not so little anymore!"
Bob is still a smashing lad who always stops by when he's at Redcar races. He may only have ten minutes but he always calls in. He has never forgotten his friends.
Margaret Neesham, nee Silman

Ha! I'd forgotten about my cooking bananas, I loved a banana ome-lette. I do still like cooking, but I think it's just as well Margaret managed to get me back into horses properly, as I don't think I'm quite a Cordon-Bleu Chef.

I was getting better at riding and my confidence was building, but I still didn't have what it took to jump. Until one day a girl in school, whose pony wouldn't jump a thing, asked me for help. I had recently met David Anker, a farmer's son who was employed as Dad's second whipper-in on the hunt. He was older than me and sort of looked out for me. He also encouraged me to ride and would help me when I was struggling. Well, David was there that day and when the girl asked me to help I thought, despite my nerves, I'd sort it out for her. I know it was all showing off and bravado, but it was just the courageous boost I needed to follow David straight over a five-barred gate. The pony jumped it effortlessly and more to the point, I stayed on. I was so pleased with myself I turned around and jumped it twice more. That was that. I was hooked. Completely crazy about riding and especially jumping. It was like someone had flicked a switch. I went from being scared of jumping fences to wanting to jump anything. I owe a lot to the pretty girl and her pony.

You could also say that the experience kicked off another trait. You couldn't stop me from being attracted to pretty girls and showing off in front of them. I think I still do to this day.

I also owe a lot to Mr McKenzie, my form-master at second-ary school. I will admit that the school 'seasons' were all wrong for me. I wanted to be off riding and hunting in the winter, but we got all the holidays in the summer, so I may have taken a few… some… well, okay, a lot of Mondays and Thursdays off. Mr McKenzie knew from the first day he met me at age eleven, that I was destined to be a jockey and he never once tried to dissuade me.

So, when I would rock up on a Tuesday or a Friday with a forged letter saying, 'Poor Bobby had the flu again...' he would pull me to one side and ask me what sort of a day I'd actually had and did I have any tips for Saturday. Thanks to him and his 'creative' marking of the register, when it came to the end of term report cards, I was often the only kid that had never had a day off all year. What a great man and I know he was so chuffed for me when I finally did become a jockey.

But I couldn't take every day off school, so I had to figure out ways to make things less boring. I certainly had to get out of my least favourite subject, physics. I can't quite remember exactly how I managed it, but I know that I ended up as the school's Head Librarian. That is no small feat for a boy who never read a book. Sadly though, during each and every physics lesson there would be a crisis in 'my library' that needed my attention. I even managed to get a team of helpers and yes, they were girls. I was also in charge of collecting the fines, but I always shared them out between us. I'm not sure why I disliked physics so much, as I went on to like engineering quite a lot.

The only aspect of school I remember having a passion for was track and field. Now, I'll grant that not many looking at me would think I was school champion at pole vaulting, but I was. In fact, I was good enough for county-level and would practice every lunchtime. I also wasn't too bad as a cross-country runner and I think that kick-started my dedication to keeping fit. I'm sure whatever latent levels I built up back then stood me in good stead when I became a jockey and, despite the pole-vaulting and the cross-country, that was fast becoming what I wanted to be.

In one way it was the only potential for what I saw as escape. I remember the careers officers coming into the school and telling us all about the employers in the area. Bearing in mind I was at the local secondary school, my choices were limited. For me and my school companions, it was the Dorman Long Steelworks or Skinningrove Mines. That was it. I didn't fancy either but was especially put off by the mines that wound their way down and out, five or ten miles under the sea. It was wet and there had been cave-ins.

They still used pit-ponies back then and if a pony had to be destroyed underground, my Dad or one of his whipper-ins had to go get it. I went in with them once, but only managed halfway. That was more than enough. The cramped, confined darkness was definitely not for me. Yet, isn't the world a strange old place? That mine is a popular museum and tourist attraction now. People pay to visit it.

What with my extra-curricular hunting activities and my desperation not to be a steelworker nor a miner, my desire to be a jockey became stronger and stronger. I rode more and more and, I suppose, became a better horseman. Certainly I developed my own way of riding.

Derek says that my riding style developed because we would both ride out in the hunts immediately behind my Dad. Like I said, he was a phenomenal horseman and when he was out in the country, hacking along and taking his horse over the various fences and obstacles, we would be tucked in behind, following his every move. I can never be accused of being the most flamboyant or indeed stylish of jockeys, but I think Derek is right. I learnt how to get the best from a horse, how to get across an obstacle, how to keep the horse moving along, even how to trick it into thinking it was travelling better than it was, all by watching my Dad during those hunts.

I suppose I did become a bit of a daredevil as time progressed. I remember Howard, Derek and I were given some cheap old motorbikes that we were allowed to ride in the fields. The deal was if we could ride them safely in there, then we might be allowed to take them onto the roads. I very quickly wrote mine off. Then Howard followed suit. Derek managed a bit better but he didn't see any roads either. But, we kept fixing them up and riding them for a couple of years and for some reason, I was the one who did the majority of the repairs. I became quite the mechanic! Of course it didn't matter how good I was at fixing them, they still needed petrol to run and we didn't have any money, so I may have… siphoned a little petrol from the cars of the people visiting the kennels. Allegedly… Howard does remember a time I swallowed a mouthful and passed out. I should add that he and Derek were very worried. Not about me, but that my Dad would come out and catch us!

I can remember that we had a significant day on the 9th December 1960. It was then that we got electricity for the first time and a TV! I can be positive it was on that day as the very first airing of Coronation Street was the first thing we watched as a family. It was also the first time in my life I went to bed without a candle. It's funny the things that stick in your mind when you look back.

Given that I would fight with Mary all the time and she was smaller than me, it was ironic that the one thing I didn't like was a bully. I remember one day coming home with a black eye. I was asked about it but wouldn't say why or what it was from. My Dad never pressed it and I thought it had long been forgotten, but years later my Dad told me he had found out from a friend that I had sorted out three bullies at school. It was strange that all those years later, it gave me such satisfaction to realise my Father had been proud of me for doing that.

As well as the hunt, Howard, Derek and I had a real passion for wrestling. We'd scrimp together as much money as we could and head off to Farrer Stadium in Middlesbrough. It wasn't really the place for 12-year olds to be and you had to pluck up all your courage to walk the streets there, but we loved the wrestling and at that age we felt we could take on the world, so a few Middlesbrough streets were nothing. If we could afford it, we'd pay for the 1/- seat, or if not you could get standing room for 6d. Of course once the house lights went down no one knew what you'd paid and we'd find ourselves better seats in the 2/6d section!

We loved the wrestler Norman Walsh, whose daughter was in our pony club, but our favourite was Masambula, a giant of a man who fought under the tag of 'The King of Charisma' and dressed as a Zulu warrior. In the early days he'd appeared in a tribal grass skirt, but after it had been set on fire by misguided fans he'd taken to wearing a full-length leopard skin. The announcer would introduce him in a great building crescendo, "From the deepest darkest Africa..." and there would always be some wise-cracker who'd shout, "No he's not, he's from down our street!" Some of the audience were funnier than the wrestling. It was so sad when Masambula, a man who had brought so much entertainment to wrestling, was badly injured in a televised bout. He ended his days in a wheelchair.

Between horses and friends and Mary, I had a pretty good childhood. Like I say, I never really cared for school that much although, what with the bikes, and despite the physics, I seemed to have an aptitude for engineering subjects.

My 'uncle' Jim (actually a friends of my fathers but whom we called uncle) was a head lad at the Royal trainer, Major Peter Cazalet's yard and Mary had been down there quite a few summers riding out. I used to go down for the summers as well and I really wanted to be taken on as an apprentice, but Jim was a hard man. He said, "No chance. We're practically related and I'd have to be harder on you than on any of the other lads."

I suppose I could see where he was coming from, but it was disappointing. Interestingly, Mary was the only girl they ever let ride in those stables, which tells you a great deal about her abilities as a jockey even at that age. It was such a prestigious yard because the Queen Mother kept her horses there and would often pop in. Mary was called on by the stable lads to polish the brasses before Her Majesty arrived, but they paid her and I don't think she minded too much.

By now, aged fifteen, I definitely knew that all I wanted to be was a jockey. However, my Dad and I were having a bit of a rough time of it. It was that all too familiar tale of a teenage son and his father having a few fall outs, it happened then and still happens now. I didn't have any inclination to do well at school and both Mum and Dad thought there might be a better opportunity for me down south.

So, in the autumn of 1963 I was sent south to Wiltshire and a job on my Uncle (my real Uncle) Arthur's farm. It was a huge culture shock to a very shy young man, stripped of family and friends in one fell swoop. That's not to say I wasn't with family, but my uncle was a dour, serious man and my Auntie Eileen wasn't as good a cook as my Mum. I used to think she could ruin any meal, but she could bake; I'll give her that. Sadly, her cakes couldn't change the reality of a young man surrounded by old people. It was therefore a bit of a relief that I was also to attend the Trowbridge Technical

College for an Engineering Diploma, but my real attraction for the job was that Uncle Arthur and Auntie Eileen always had at least one point-to-point horse in training each season. Saying that, by the end of my college course I did graduate with an Engineering Diploma and 'O' levels in English, Maths and History. I was quite chuffed with myself.

During that time money was still tight and more often than not I'd just walk to the college. It was only a few miles and the exercise did me good. It also meant I got there at about the same time as the bus, what with its meandering route. Thing is, you could claim your bus fares back, so I would always pick up a discarded ticket next to the last stop. The extra few quid at the end of term was always welcome.

Strangely, after my lack of interest in school, I really did enjoy the college environment and the engineering. I remember the final exam was to put an engine back together, a thing I did relatively easily. So I was okay at it, but I remember truly loving the farming. Well, I loved driving tractors and ploughing. I wasn't as keen on hoeing and still wasn't a fan of cows.

But of course, the horse riding was my main incentive in being down there. Though it wasn't a free ride. The days were hard. I'd be in the farmyard by six, mucking out the two or three horse boxes, saddling up one of the horses, exercising it for an hour or so, then breakfast and on the bus, or walking, to college. Study engineering all day, then back to the farm, dress over the horses, feed them, do other odd jobs, then bed. But on a Saturday, in the winter months, I got to go hunting and I knew I was improving all the time. Although, the first official ride I had on my Uncle's horse, Holmcourt, a small eleven-year-old mare, wasn't a great indicator of future success.

φ

It was February 1964 and I was saddling up in a proper point-to-point. Glad all Over by the Dave Clark Five was No.2 in the charts and I came up to the last fence with a bit of a chance, but I was a touch too keen and pushed him too hard. The horse fell and I was instantly anything but glad all over. I hit the ground very, very hard, picked myself up, counted the bruises and thought, 'This isn't the game for me.' Mary, who had come to watch and had been so excited at the prospect of her big brother being in a proper race, remembers feeling very upset for me, but probably not as upset as I was!

Despite that, a month later, I rode Holmcourt again, in the Tedworth Adjacent Hunts race at Larkhill and for the first time in a proper race, I won. I truly was glad all over. The feeling was, and still is, a strange one to explain. I was happy, yes, but it was more than that. It certainly wasn't the adulation of the crowd, as you could probably have counted the spectators on both hands, but the sense of accomplishment, the sense of beating the other horses and riders. The sense that I had put everything I had learnt until then into practice and done it as well as I could. It gave me a buzz and a thrill like nothing I had ever experienced before. It was terrific, fantastic. I think the crux of my feelings, and perhaps the seeds of any professional sportsperson, is the desire to win. The need to win, regardless of prize or onlookers. It's a competitive spirit, but enhanced, amplified. It isn't just a 'want to', it's a 'need to.' What I distinctly remember is knowing that I had found the thing I should be doing. Although looking at some of the old photos from that day, I do look like a bit of a cowboy. In fact, I look at them nowadays and wonder how on earth I ever made it as a jockey.

Next time out I fell again, but in the April, I won for the second time in the Craven Farmers race at Lockinge. That was a real 'Champion Day' as my cousin Billy won the Open race on Domaboy. My four races on that little mare, Holmcourt, had settled any lingering doubts I might have had. I was fifteen and I knew I was going to be a professional jockey. I wanted to start on that right away, but a number of connections to my father said that I should take my time. Ride more amateur races. Build up to it.

I therefore finished my time at Trowbridge College, gained my Engineering Diploma and spent the next three years working on the farm for my Uncle. All that while I stayed riding in point-to-points. I remember one horse called Gipsy Melody. She was a great prospect, owned by my Uncle and she did win a few races, but respiratory problems stopped her short at times. Nonetheless, she was a really sound jumper who would gain ground at every obstacle. I reckon I was a might too brave back then, but at the time she was my ideal partner, yet often when we wanted to quicken at the end of a race she'd gurgle, like she couldn't get a breath. We were a great combination, though fair's fair, when our Mary rode her she was even better. My little sister really was a good rider. She took it as far as she could back then, but if she'd been riding now, I don't think anything would have stopped her from becoming one of the best jockeys in the country, male or female.

I did learn a lot about being a jockey in those years. I also knocked off some rough edges and over-confident corners. I can remember riding at Larkhill against David Maundrell. He was on a top-class hunter-chaser called Lizzy the Lizard and my Uncle had told me not to leave it late. I thought I knew better and figured I'd leave it until after the last, then ride it out to a win. David and I went over the last neck and neck, but, just like my Uncle had reckoned, Lizzy the Lizard was far stronger on the run-in. I recall being really, really angry at myself for not having listened. I know that from then on, all the way through my career, I tried hard not to make the same mistake twice.

During those seasons I had met Peter Calver. He was a gentle giant of a man, yet he always managed to make the weight for the local point-to-points. I knew him as a vet, farmer and trainer, but also as the owner of a great horse, Highland Wedding. He'd won a few races on him, but then he sold him to a friend of his, the trainer Toby Balding. I'll tell you what happened to the horse later, but for now, Peter kept telling me I was too good for point-to-points and that I should talk to Toby and get a job with him. Now, I'm not sure if Peter just wanted to get rid of me because I used to beat him regularly in our point-to-point clashes, but thanks to his introduction, Toby told me there was a job waiting for me if I wanted it.

If I'm honest, I had outgrown my Auntie Eileen and Uncle Arthur's yard. I mean I loved it there, but the farm was quite isolated and a lack of transport options was definitely curtailing any social life I was trying to get on with, like any young man of the time. I was by now turning nineteen, it was the summer of love and if I wanted a date it meant getting a bus to the Trowbridge cinema. It was hardly the 'Swinging Sixties' for me.

The isolation and the fact there weren't that many horses in the yard, which meant I couldn't ride as much as I wanted, made the decision easier than it might have been. So, in August 1967, I joined Toby Balding as an amateur jockey and was given a nominal role of 'Farm Manager' that would help to justify my amateur status.

Toby came from an impressive racing dynasty. His father, who had been in charge of a polo team in the US when Toby was born, later went on to train back in England. Toby's younger brother Ian trained the legendary 1971 Derby winner Mill Reef. His nephew Andrew, would go on to win the Oaks in 2003 with Casual Look. Ian's daughter, and Toby's niece, Clare Balding is the renowned television presenter. Over a career that lasted almost fifty years Toby won over 2,000 races and notably completed the treble of the Gold Cup, the Champion Hurdle (twice) and the Grand National (twice). He was also responsible for fostering the careers of riders such as Richard Linley, Adrian Maguire, AP McCoy... and me I suppose.

His yard was famous for keeping as many jockeys as horses, but because I could claim the weight allowance of an inexperienced jockey, he said I'd get race rides and that was good enough for me. I had made it. I was a jockey. I was delighted, but that delight only lasted a day. On the second morning in the yard, things went very badly wrong.

φ

I was given a leg-up onto a horse called Dozo, a handicap chaser who had only just come back into training after a summer out at grass. I should have factored that in and been a lot more cautious, but the Guv'nor asked me to ride it out and I was new. I took hold of Dozo's reins, threw my leg over and landed down on his back. The horse, unused to a weight on him, reared up, fell backwards and pinned me on the ground. I heard the bones in my ankle and foot snap with a noise like a gunshot.

I couldn't believe it. Not only had I broken my ankle, but the break was so bad, so complex, that it took a week for the swelling to subside enough for the surgeons to sort things out. I still have the pins in me to this day. The only good thing to come out of it was meeting Mrs Mita Easton. She was the anaesthetist on the operation, but she was also a rider, a trainer and owned a pub. What a lady! She'd been born in the 1920's, was left a horse in a will in 1945 and it was even later when she decided to start riding in point-to-points. As she was putting me under she promised me that she would send a couple of rides my way, and she did. Apparently she thought I was a 'lovely horseman' and I couldn't help but like her eccentric way of ringing me at five in the morning to book me.

When finally allowed out of hospital I went back to Toby's yard and worked in the office until my foot was mended. Eventually, at the end of October, I got my first opportunity to ride a race as a proper amateur jockey. The horse was a novice called Swiss Knight and the track was Worcester, over fences. After a mile we were so far behind that I pulled him up. It was an inauspicious start. Still, next time out at Fontwell we started at 66-1 in a seven horse race and to my delight and surprise, we came third.

Toby also had a horse called Altercation. It was well named and made Swiss Knight look like Arkle. No one wanted to ride it, not even me, because it had fallen every time it had run, be it over hurdles or steeplechase fences. For whatever reason, best known to himself, Toby decided to run it and Swiss Knight together at Plumpton. Clive Bailey got the ride on Altercation and I got Swiss Knight. We both knew we didn't stand a chance, but Clive and myself decided to have a side bet to see who could go furthest. I shot away to an early lead, then fell back like I knew I would and Clive passed me by, all smiles. When he fell at the next fence I remember grinning down at him as he lay in the mud. I managed to get Swiss Knight over one more fence before I pulled him up.

I learnt other things whilst at Toby's and one of those was, I don't like to drink to excess! This may have had something to do with the very first night I went out with the other young jockeys. We went to the local pub and they decided to play 'Spoofing', which is a game of chance to figure out who buys the next round.

It turns out I was very good at it and before long I had fifteen Newcastle Brown Ales lined up on the bar. I can't quite remember how many I managed to put away before chucking out time, but it was a lot. I was up all night being sick, then was sick in the morning getting ready for work, then sick again out on the gallops and sick again each and every time I mucked out one of the stables. Oh was I sick and I vowed, like every young fella after his first horrendous hangover, that I would, 'never again.' The difference was for me, it stuck and whilst I've enjoyed a drink in my time, it was rarely again to excess!

I also bought my first car. I saved up £90 for a green and black Mini I bought off an old butcher. I thought it was a cracker of a car and she never let me down. It also meant that I had a certain amount of freedom and I think this finally spurred on my interest in the opposite sex. I've got to admit, I was never as interested in cars as women, but I do have very fond memories of that old Mini. My next car was a Hillman Imp and my goodness what a pile of rubbish that was! Always breaking down on me.

On the 21st November 1967, I finished second at Fontwell on the mare Last Town, owned and trained by the lovely anaesthetist, Mrs Easton and I was really getting into the whole swing of things when for the first time in its history, the Jockey Club suspended racing in its entirety. It was legitimately in response to a Foot and Mouth epidemic that was sweeping the nation and had already led to the mass slaughter of millions of farm animals, but that didn't lessen the impact on racing. I remember everyone was miserable, me included, but at least it gave my ankle even more time to heal and strengthen. Racing was stopped from the 25th November to the 5th January. It then resumed for two days before bad weather stopped it for another ten days. I could feel my frustration and everyone else's mounting.

Eventually, the weather cleared, racing was resumed all over the country and I was given the task of nursing the dangerous Altercation around Plumpton in another novice chase. I was fairly underwhelmed at the prospect if I'm honest. Being dumped onto the ground by a handful of a horse hardly seemed like a fun thing to do, but the Guv'nor said I was riding it so that was that. Truth is, I was still super keen and would have taken a ride on anything.

I know we started at odds of 20-1, but no one in their right mind would have backed him at 200s. To be fair, he wasn't the ideal mount for someone as inexperienced as I was, but my enthusiasm made up for a lack of ability and the absence of fear. I also believe that if you really want to be a jump jockey then at the start of your career you have to take the unpredictable and dangerous mounts. Those horses that the older heads around the game would avoid. The 'Dodgy Rides' that could seriously give you problems. It's how you learn.

I can recall everyone in the yard saying the horse would 'bury me' and they were betting on just how long I'd manage to stay upright. I wasn't exactly looking forward to the race but it turned out that we were all wrong. Altercation picked his feet up, jumped well, three fences out we hit the front and won nicely. I thought I was God's gift to racing. Sadly, on my next two outings on him he promptly fell in short order, so maybe I wasn't quite as good as I thought.

In fact, it was the next time out on him, again back at Plumpton, which resulted in me having my first serious concussion. Altercation ploughed his way through several fences like he thought it was his mission to demolish them and at the ninth, fell heavily. I woke up in the ambulance room and then later in the hospital, suffering from severe concussion. The thing is, I checked myself out of the hospital that night, but didn't get back home until six in the morning. Quite seriously, from that day to this, I have no idea where I was in those intervening hours. I know racing was different then, I understand it was a different time and a different mentality, but the concussions we suffered and how we coped with them were something not really discussed or dealt with. Thankfully, it is a far cry from nowadays when jockeys are looked after far more rigorously than we ever were. Or perhaps the system has become so much better at protecting jockeys from their biggest worst enemy, themselves.

Back in 1968, I shook off the concussion and went on to have a number of winners in those early months. More so, I began to get a feel for the racing game. I learnt the ropes of what I needed to be and I discovered a few things about myself as a jockey.

The truth is, horses don't have much in the way of consistency. Each one is different, each one an individual, so you have to get used to them and as an amateur or professional 'riding-under-rules' jockey, you have to get used to them quickly. Find out their temperament. Judge their ability. Try to get the feel of them. It's one of the strange things about horse racing that for probably half of the rides I had, I'd never sat on the horse before the paddock. A lot of non-racing people don't realise that, but we accepted it as part of the job. Compare that to any other sport, where the competitor has been using the same equipment, or playing with the same team mates, practising, getting familiar, learning all their idiosyncrasies, for months, maybe even years. Not for the jockey and their mount. Time to discover each other could be less than five minutes. But I loved it. It was the mark of the professional that I wanted to be.

And you weren't on your own. You were always chatting to the other jockeys. One of them might have ridden it before and they'd tell you any quirks worth knowing. The lad or lass leading you out would tell you something about its attitude that morning and the Guv'nor, the trainer, would tell you something else. So out of all that, you had to put everything together. Then it was up and into the saddle and cantering down to the start. I found that I could get a good feeling for the horse then. Be able to pick it up. Know if it was well-balanced, if it liked the ground. Or not.

Of course, there was the odd occasion when you thought, 'Oh, this isn't going to be good. This thing could hurt me.' But you had to get on with it.

I discovered a love for Ascot, Sandown, Newbury, Plumpton, Fontwell and the beautiful, but dangerous, little Wye. I dreamt of Cheltenham and Aintree.

I also found that I didn't like using the whip that much. I discovered that I could 'kid' a horse into believing it was going better than it was. You may ask, 'how do you kid a horse?' Well you just keep taking a pull, and squeezing, keeping them thinking it's going well. Keeping their rhythm. It sounds strange, but it used to work much better for me than giving them a crack with the whip, when some of the horses would just curl up.

As that first year wound on, I also realised that I was going to have to deal with a few personal issues. Toby for instance, outside of work was a warm, friendly and fun-loving man, and I wouldn't hear anyone say anything other than that about him. He had a steady temperament and a kind personality, but in the yard or on the course he wasn't shy of bawling you out if he thought you needed it. Given his track record and his legacy, his methods were obviously effective, but that whole approach didn't really work for me.

If I had a fancied ride, Toby would start niggling me first thing in the morning out on the gallops. He wouldn't leave it all day. I know some people who ride better when they're wound up, but I'm definitely not one of them. I always felt more confident in a race if I thought he wasn't watching and I did feel that win or lose, Toby seemed to give me a bollocking regardless. It demoralised me. I'm sure he didn't mean it, and I'm sure it worked for many another jockey, but for me, well to be honest, I found it quite depressing.

However, the main realisation I had during those early months, and something that was to be a constant struggle throughout my career; was my weight. In old-fashioned terms, I'm what's described as five-foot-nine, thick-set, and big-boned. And, I enjoy my food. Well, who doesn't? I would, on occasion, rather miss meals and have ice cream and chocolate bars, then think I could sweat it all off in the sauna. The truth is I could. I became a sauna master.

During my time as a jockey I have calculated that I spent twenty-three hours per racing season week, every year for ten years in a sauna. That's just over 10,000 hours so that must make me an expert! My routine was well practised. I would have half a small cup of coffee to warm me up inside and then cover myself in baby oil. Baby oil is very good as it works in two ways, one it allows you to get hot without having the sauna turned up to maximum and two, it stops the sweat from going back into your pores. There'd always be several jockeys in there, and especially in the later years in the sauna in Hungerford, which in my opinion was the best, we'd often take bets to see who could fill up a glass of sweat the fastest! Well, it was such a boring place, you couldn't read anything as the paper got soggy, so we'd just sit around and moan about what a stupid job we had. Extreme sauna was for when you were struggling to shift that last pound. You'd turn the sauna right up, stick your head in a bucket of cold water until you had to come up for breath. Looking back now I know it sounds ridiculous, but it was the only thing we knew that worked and a race could depend on that last pound. One of the sure facts in the whole of racing was and is, that one pound of weight meant one length of distance and that could mean the difference between first and nowhere.

We (the dedicated sauna jockey club) always tried to meet every Sunday at 4pm, but looking back, my efforts at fasting and wasting and sweating were erratic, unhealthy and probably dangerous. Soon I was introduced to Diuretics or what were colloquially known as 'Piss Pills'. One of them could cause you to lose a few pounds rapidly through peeing, but the side effects could be devastating. In those early days, again a different time and a different mentality to the standards of today, I would use them as a last resort. As a short-term measure they did seem ideal, but I soon found that I would put on twice as much weight in the evening as I had lost in the morning. Sometimes I felt so weak after taking them that I was literally nothing more than a passenger on the horse. Also, if you had a fall whilst on them you'd certainly know about it as you really felt the ground when you landed. You hurt far more than when you weren't taking them.

The lack of medical oversight back then probably didn't do us many favours at all and the modern jockey, better looked after, better educated and frankly, much less likely to take the risks we took, are so much more capable of regulating their weight through diet control and exercise. They also have other advantages, such as better technology, the saddles are much lighter and they're given equipment allowances. I'd say that they've probably gained a 3lb advantage on my contemporaries. A full 3lb is a huge difference, especially for instance, if I needed to be weighing out at 10st 6lb, then because our kit weighed 4lb at least, my weight had to be 10st 2lb or less. That was a hard ask.

So, we often had to go to extreme measures and we'd have cheating-boots where they barely had a sole on and were incredibly light, just for the weigh out. I was often targeted for coming in heavier than I went out. Some of this could be attributed to rain absorption, yes this did happen, particularly if you'd taken Diuretics as the body needed the moisture, but also it could be down to sodden colours and mud. Of course some of it was down to careful balancing of the scales. We were all very good at getting the best weight and it became a game and a thrill for us. There was never any malice or any intention to cheat and a lot of the clerks of the scales would help you out. If you went to see them and explained you'd struggled that week, then they'd help you with the odd few ounces.

But, there was always that one 'job's worth' that would 'kick-off'. That's how the story of my heavy cup of tea after the 1977 Hennessy Gold Cup came about! But we'll get to that later.

The Major
I've mentioned the problems I had with my weight, but in the 'good old days' the clerk of the scales who looked after the weighing room were mostly flexible and understanding. But, sometimes you could get one or two that were a little annoying. Then there was 'The Major'.

He and I didn't see eye-to-eye on most things and our relationship was a little fractious. He was a former Army Major and I think it was perhaps his officious manner that used to rub me up the wrong way. I do remember putting a piss pill into his tea on one occasion at a meeting, but it was at Sandown that everything came to a head. Almost literally.

I'd done my weight and won the race. Then I came back into the weighing room and my weight was different by half a pound. Given the exertions of the ride, that was nothing. Perfectly normal, but he kept on and on and on.

I can clearly remember lifting my racing helmet and

swinging my arm back to launch it at his head. But as my arm reached its full backswing, Jeff King, who had just come in and was walking behind me, casually took the helmet out of my hand.

Later I said thank you to Jeff.

"No problem, Bob, I knew what you were going to do and they'd have banned you for life."

He was right, but oh I had been so wild. That Major knew just how to wind me up.

Yet all the rest of the clerks of the scales were so much more fun. I think all of that mischief has probably gone from the modern game as things are a lot more regulated.

By mid-April 1968 I had ridden eight winners and was fourth in the amateur jockey list behind the leader, Richard Tate. The way amateur status worked back then was that the Jockey Club would interview you after a set number of wins, or a set number of races. Usually, they waited for you to have ten winners, then the licensing stewards would interview you, verify your amateur status and issue you with a B-class permit. I was interviewed after about forty-five rides, still two short of my tenth winner. What I thought would be a fairly casual chat took place in London on the 20th April, and it lasted fifteen long, long minutes. I was asked over and over to explain how I could afford to continue riding as an amateur. I explained my position as Toby's Farm Manager. The licensing steward wasn't convinced.

"So... Farm Manager, eh? What exactly do you do?" he asked with not a little incredulousness.

"I look after the gallops," I answered, eager to show my knowledge of all things Farm Manager.

"And what do you do, on the gallops?"

"Mow them..." Even I thought that was a bit light, so I added, "And tread in the divots."

"What else do you do on the farm?" asked another steward.

Basically, by this time I was struggling. I offered, "Ummm, I collect the eggs?"

"And just how many chickens does Mr Balding keep?" said the first steward with his eyebrow raised in amazed anticipation.

"Ummm, five?... I think."

I wouldn't have been convinced either. The stewards definitely weren't. They ruled I had been riding and working for payment and that was an infringement of my amateur status. In a really unusual turn of events, they withdrew my licence to ride completely. I was mortified. The whole affair dragged on for two weeks. I honestly began to wonder if that was my career over before it began. Toby was livid with the authorities. So much so that he went to the Jockey Club in Newmarket and appealed the decision. Eventually, in early May, the stewards relented and I was issued with a professional licence. Now, given that I wanted to be a jockey, you may think that sounds like the answer to all my dreams, but at the time it was the last thing I wanted. I honestly didn't think I was good enough to be offered paid rides yet. It meant mixing it with the professionals and I was far from confident. But it all turned out all right I guess. Although I still can't look at a box of chicken eggs without smiling.

So it was that on the 13th May 1968, after an absence from the track of almost a month, I rode again for Toby Balding, but this time, for the first time, as a professional jockey. The horse was Sailor's Collar and the track was the tight and treacherous Wye. That wonderful track has long ago closed because of the amount of fallers and injuries it had, but I loved the place. In fact, I was the leading jockey at the course for several seasons. If you went round Wye and gave up the outside to nobody, you would always gain ground because the horse would always be balanced. I'll admit it was dangerous when it rained and there would be a lot of fallers on the bends, but I wish we still raced there. I think my love for the track started that day in May 1968. That first professional ride on Sailor's Collar, and that moment when we won in style.

Being a professional jockey, like all walks of life, came with its own quirks and foibles. The changing room experience being the main one. On your professional debut you'd be assigned a changing room peg. It was a simple, yet traditional system. The new jockey got the peg nearest the door. As the older hands retired, or sadly died, the jockeys would move to the next peg along.

So it was that for all of my professional career I would have Bob Davies in front and Bill Smith behind.

As well as your peg, you needed a valet, but you didn't get to pick them. They chose you. Back then being a valet was a generational, family thing. I think it was Dick Francis that said it was the ultimate closed shop. There were about half a dozen families, that through the fathers and sons and brothers, cousins and uncles would provide the services to all the jockeys up and down the country. They looked after everything from boots to helmets, sweaters to saddles, all of it taken away at the end of the day and made ready again for the next. It meant all I had to do was turn up at the course.

As well as all of that, they were like the ultimate golfing caddy, counsellor and personal dresser all rolled into one. They'd know what horse you were riding and the weight you were meant to be, so they'd supply all the proper kit, from a heavy or light saddle to the extra lead needed to bring a lighter jockey up to weight. As well as that, they'd listen to you after a race and if you'd been banged about in a fall they'd help get you ready for the next. They were, and remain, an essential yet little seen part of racing.

The man who chose to look after me from my first day was known as 'Pipe-smoking Robin'. He was amazing. In a job that was immensely busy and hectic, looking after half a dozen or more jockeys at a time, he never appeared rushed or stressed, yet everything was always done. No task was too difficult. He was like the proverbial swan. All calm and grace on the surface but he must have been working very, very hard underneath. He could also read me like a book.

As the years progressed he'd see me coming in after a lousy ride and know that my pent up frustration would have me throwing the saddle across the room. He invariably caught it, laughed at me and in an instant my frustration and anger would be gone. Then, without a word, he would set about getting me ready for the next race.

Many years after my debut, Robin would make the journey to Aintree in April 1981, even though he didn't have to, just to be there for me on that very special day.

And They're Off

Without much of a break, for the next eleven years, I would be a professional jockey, both in the UK and in America. It was my dream come true, albeit it would have its ups and downs. One of the early ups was riding a Grand National winner in my very first professional season, just not in the National itself.

In February 1969, the twelve-year-old Highland Wedding, once the property of that gentle giant Peter Calver, but now owned by an American partnership, was sent north to Newcastle for the Eider Chase and I was to be his jockey.

I'd ridden him before, three months earlier at Chepstow and we'd finished third. A good result considering the horse had shown little form in the previous year. I'd been given that ride because his regular jockey, Owen McNally, was out of action with an injury. Given that I'd got him in the frame, I had high hopes of riding him again, but next time out I was replaced by the brilliant Irish horseman, Eddie Harty and he and Highland Wedding won. However, neither Harty nor McNally were available for the Eider, so I was called back again.

On the morning of the race, Toby was insistent that I not come a cropper and get unseated as I had done when on Time is Money the previous day at Kempton. He spread out the morning papers, which had a photograph of me sailing through the air, and forcefully told me he did not expect a repeat.

"Be careful, Bob. No heroics at the last."

I remember walking the course twice. It was soft, almost heavy, testing conditions but Highland Wedding started out as favourite as he had won the same race in '66 and '67 and probably would have done it in '68 as well, had the meeting not been cancelled for bad weather.

We set off and I rode a patient race, moved easily into the lead with a mile left and approaching the last, I had it won. All I had to do was get over the fence. All I nearly did was blow it. We'd jumped brilliantly all the way round, but, because I had Toby's warning playing loud in my head, I was concentrating way too much on being careful. I'd been giving Highland Wedding a kick into all the fences, but this time I was motionless. He got much too close, clattered the top, arched his back and landed steeply. I never really thought I'd come off, but it made for an exciting spectacle for any punters who had backed him. We went on to win easily and following the victory, Highland Wedding was lined up for a third, and what would be his last, attempt at the Grand National.

I heard Toby describe me as 'a natural horseman' to a bunch of reporters so I hoped I might retain the ride, but they gave it back to the much more experienced Harty. He was a truly magnificent jockey, so I couldn't argue with the logic of it. Sure enough, that April as I watched on TV back at Fyfield, Highland Wedding and Eddie Harty drew clear of the field and won the 1969 Grand National by twelve lengths. I felt a little conflicted. Obviously I was delighted for the horse and all its connections, but I couldn't help thinking, 'what if?' Although, if I'm totally honest, I'd probably not have been experienced enough to do him justice at Liverpool, having never ridden there. But it would have been nice to have had the chance.

They did give him back to me to ride in the Midlands National at Uttoxeter in the May, but two fences in I knew he was beaten. Any horse that competes at Aintree has run a hard race even if they don't show outward signs of it. The winner usually the hardest of all. I was on a hiding to nothing at Uttoxeter, the old horse was tired from the get go, so I pulled him up as soon as I could.

φ

I finished my first professional season with fifteen winners, which I thought was a perfectly respectable score. Especially given that Toby had so many jockeys in the yard and the competition to get rides was always fierce. On that point, competition was fierce between all the professionals, but the thing I loved most about being a jockey was the sense of belonging to an exclusive, yet tightly knit club. We were bound by the shared experiences, the shared risks. We were all competitive, we all wanted the ride, we all wanted the win, yet I can honestly testify that there was never any malice, animosity or jealousy within the yards, or in the changing or weighing rooms. Each of us tried our hardest, there is no question about that, but as soon as our race was over, win or lose, we were reunited with our 'family'. More often than not we would almost all go out together after the races and we had each other's backs. Even when the time came to hang up my riding boots for good, that common bond, that sense of special kinship, never diminished between the jockeys. I loved it. I still do.

So my first full year as a pro had been alright, but the next few years were to prove how hard the racing game could be. You see when you're an amateur and even when still a novice professional, you get a weight allowance to make up for your inexperience. Like I said before, a pound weight is a length's advantage and it makes a massive difference. That's why some of the French authorities were up in arms at the end of 2017 concerning the granting of weight allowances for female jockeys. Although I can't blame the likes of Hayley Turner for taking advantage of it. I know I would have. I certainly did back when I was a novice and when I lost it, after my twenty-fifth win, I had to compete on level terms with the best of them. Of course Toby still had quite a lot of young jockeys able to claim allowances, so he used them to his full advantage. It meant getting rides became harder. However, I continued to work as a stable lad, up at dawn, mucking out several horses, exercising at least three of them, then back and grooming three or four of them until six in the evening. And all the time hoping for races.

Of course with fewer rides my earnings dropped, but I did manage to scrape together enough for my first brand new car. It was a Fiat and whilst I thought it was impressive, sadly it was anything but. It really was quite a dreadful car and in damp weather it simply wouldn't start. You'd have to take half the wires out to dry them just to get it going. Although I wasn't to know that straight away. In fact I wasn't to know that until I got its replacement, because the first time I drove this one, I had a bit more of an issue to contend with.

It was the very first car I had ever picked up new from a garage and feeling as proud as punch, I drove off to a waiting ride at Nottingham races. I'd only been in it fifteen minutes when I rounded a bend to see a stationary Land Rover, with a trailer hitched to it, sitting smack bang on my side of the road. There was nowhere for me to go except into it, which I did, hard.

The force shoved the engine block back into my knee and I was trapped in the car. Had that engine come a further two inches back, I'd have lost my leg from the knee down. As it was I never made it to Nottingham and I was out of racing for nearly two months.

Six months later in the second version of the car, my rising damp replacement Fiat and I were taking a girlfriend home when I hit a patch of black ice. The sad little car which couldn't really go that fast, managed to hit a curb, flip up and over a brick wall and threw in a double somersault. My girlfriend went through the windscreen and I was thrown into the back of the car.

I know that there is good reason for them now, but back in the 1970's seatbelts weren't compulsory. In this instance it's a good job we hadn't been wearing them or both my girlfriend and I would have been dead. The front end of the car was completely flattened and needless to say it was a total write off. We both ended up in hospital and thankfully, apart from scrapes and bruises, we were both fine. I was given the task of ringing her Dad, who promptly banned me from seeing his daughter again. I guess I can understand it, but it was a shame as she was very pretty. I decided to give up on Fiats after that and bought a Datsun.

What with the lack of rides and the time off with the first car accident, by the end of the season in June 1970, I had only ridden ten winners. I did wonder if I shouldn't have stuck with Uncle Arthur and Auntie Eileen on the farm. It's strange how confidence is such a fragile thing in professional sportspeople. You begin to doubt yourself and your abilities. Like a football striker who isn't getting the goals. It can become a vicious circle. Then you realise it is only you feeling sorry for yourself. You shake yourself out of it and keep going. Nothing else to be done for it.

So, being young and resilient, I went off on a summer break with a new girlfriend and returned in July, tanned and ready to attack the new season, confidence renewed. Two days before the opening meeting I was legged-up onto a novice chaser called Pieces who had just been brought in from a summer at grass. Now, I have said earlier that I tried hard to learn from my every mistake. You may remember that I had jumped up on a novice chaser brought in from a summer at grass before and it hadn't ended well. You'd think I'd have remembered. But, it turns out, not so much.

On the very same spot where I had broken my ankle three years previously, Pieces went berserk, reared up, I went out the back and as I was regaining my feet, the horse kicked, shattering my left ankle. I was in plaster and out of action for months and have to admit I was not the happiest of chaps. In fact I was a complete boor. I put on weight, got on everyone's nerves and basically made a right nuisance of myself. There were times I felt like packing the whole thing in, but the truth is that every time I contemplated it I realised there was nothing to rival racing at speed over fences. Nothing in life that even came close. Not for me. The fact that all I wanted to do was race made each day I was injured drag like a week.

It was October before I was passed fit to ride and then I had to wait until the following January at Nottingham for my first winner on the aptly named, You're Lucky. It was my first winner in eleven months. I was moping around and feeling a bit down and then… things looked up again.

φ

I rode a small mare called Country Wedding to victory at Taunton in the March. She was a lovely, sensible little horse by the same sire as Highland Wedding and was a dour stayer. The Taunton victory prompted Toby to enter her for the National. He came to me and asked if I wanted the ride.

To try to explain what that moment felt like is very hard for me now. I was just 24½ years old. A kid. Riding in the National had been a dream of mine since I was eight. The emotions were intense. Country Wedding wasn't quick, she wasn't big and she couldn't jump, but it was a ride in the National and if I was to win, well… I just had to hope everything else would fall. It didn't matter one jot to me. I'd have ridden a clothes horse if it got me into the race. But, if I was to be the jockey, I needed to get to ten stone dead.

I did it, just, but only thanks to spending most of the week before the race in saunas, eating little and taking laxatives. I was quite chuffed. I'd not managed ten stone many times in my life. We stayed over in Chester the night before and I tried to get some sleep, but my mind was full of the images of Aintree. I got up and rode out in the morning. As for breakfast, well I think that was half a cup of coffee.

Later I walked the National course for the first time. The thing is, I'd never been to Aintree before. Not even as a spectator. Now here I was, about to ride round it. The surprising thing is the fences are not as big as you'd think… really. Or at least that's what I tried to tell myself. The logical part of my brain was screaming, 'horses can't jump these, they're massive, this is ridiculous.' Eventually, I suppressed my fear by telling myself, 'people had been jumping over them for a hundred years, so if they can, you can.' Ah, the exuberance of youth. Fence No.3, the first of the big open ditches, frightened me more than most. I can remember standing in front of this monster of an enormous, 4ft 10in high, spruce–topped fence with a huge 6ft ditch in front of it and saying over and over, 'I suppose I've jumped things as big as this when out hunting.' Then I paused before admitting, 'just not at racing pace.' As it turned out, the third fence wasn't going to cause me any issues.

The whole build up to the race is suitably big. You have a full twenty-five minutes to file out, get into the paddock, get mounted up, parade in front of the grandstands, go down to the first, then return to the start and wait for what seems to be ages for the starter to call the field forward. All that tension and tingling atmosphere builds and builds. The nerves increase. Even the most experienced jockeys are affected by it. For me, normally quiet in the preliminaries of a race, it turned me into a chatterbox.

I had no need to be nervous. I was on a 50-1 shot that was largely ignored. It was a strange feeling. I was riding in a race with no chance at all. Country Wedding didn't even jump little fences that well. There wasn't a snowball's chance that she'd win and not much of a one that she'd even get round the whole race. Toby simply told me to go out and enjoy myself. But I harboured ambitions. I thought, 'okay, we might not have a chance, but for once, I'm going to be smart. I'm going to be wise beyond my years.' I knew the little mare didn't have the speed to push the leaders, not even in the run up to the first, so I figured, if I tucked in behind a safe pair of hands, then that would be a very good idea. None safer than Terry Biddlecombe on the previous year's winner, Gay Trip. Brilliant strategy.

Thirty-eight runners, all turning and tracking around down at the start. Thirty-eight jockeys manoeuvring for best position. Well, thirty-seven and me, tracking wherever Terry went. He went wide, I went with him, he came in to line at the tapes, I tucked in behind him. He was going to be my guide and talisman. After what seemed like hours, the tapes went up, the Aintree crowd roared and we were off in the 1971 Grand National, thundering away in the long, long run to the first. A 'relatively small' fence that's only 4ft 6in high and 2ft 9in wide.

Gay Trip was just behind and to the outside of the leaders. I was right on his heels. The first wave of horses tend to hit the first fence much faster than they should, but clever me had got Country Wedding in the second wave, so was much better paced and because of that she met it perfectly. It was a great jump, I was so impressed, right up until I cleared the thick, deep green foliage of Lake District spruce and landed on the already fallen Gay Trip. One somersault later and I was fired out of the saddle like it was an ejector seat. I rolled tight, waited for the thundering hooves to pass me by and then stood up. It turned out I was in good company.

Richard Evans on Brian's Best had been brought down like myself, Peter Ennis on Craigbrook had fallen nearer the inside of the track, there was Terry on Gay Trip just beside me and Eddie Harty on Twigarairy, also brought down by Terry, just to his other side. Gay Trip had been the winning horse in 1970, Eddie the winning jockey in '69. It should have made me feel a bit better. It didn't. I was livid and heartbroken. I wanted them to stop the race. Rewind it. Start again please. I know I kept muttering, "I can't believe it," all the way back to the weighing room. That was it. My race was over. Thankfully, the camaraderie of the other jockeys came back to the fore and they were able to help raise my spirits. When, after one of the closest and most thrilling finishes in the race's history, John Cook came home victorious on Specify, I even offered a joke myself by saying, "I'd been going well up until I fell," but I was, as we'd say nowadays, truly gutted. It was so frustrating to think I'd have to wait another year for a second chance and what if no one ever wanted me to ride for them in the great race again? I mean, so far my record of one start, one fall at the first fence, was not that appealing.

It took me a while to shake the feeling of a missed opportunity and the season ended in a sort of whimper. I'd only added eight winners all year to a tally that now stood at forty-three in four years. My own dream of being in the top ten jump jockeys seemed a remote and distant goal.

But even then there were little up moments. I went off to Ostend in the summer and on Wide World I won the Prix Fabien Hurdle. Although, yet again, I'd had to work hard using extreme fasting and unhealthy methods to make the weight. I look back and wonder just how much pressure all this was putting onto my body. Was it a contributory factor to what was looming in my future? Of course, I didn't know then what I know now and I doubt it would have stopped me. I was desperate to be a top jockey. After the 70-71 season I hoped for better.

φ

Sadly, my 71-72 season wasn't.

I managed a measly ten winners, but I was given another chance in the National. I even got to have another pairing with good old Country Wedding. This time I spent the morning of the race in a sauna with a whole bunch of other jockeys. That pre-National morning sauna was to become a bit of a tradition and kept us out of the way of the press and the punters. It was also a good laugh and a great way of letting some of the big-race nerves dissipate. Regardless of it and all the other steam sessions I'd had, I couldn't make the ten stone, so carried four over into a field of forty-two runners.

It was a massive cavalry charge of horses that went off towards the Melling Road when the tapes were hoisted. Terry was there again, on Gay Trip, but I decided I'd plough my own furrow this time. We set off and I managed to stay on for the first and the second, the massive open ditch that was the third and the fourth. It's a true mark of the Grand National that if I listed the jockey royalty that fell in the '72 running at those early fences, you'd wonder how anyone ever won the race at all.

At the first, Ron Barry went alongside Tommy Stack. Ron would go on to win the Whitbread Gold Cup three times and was Champion Jockey in the '73 and '74 seasons. Tommy Stack was Champion in '75 and '77 but is best known for steering Red Rum to his third National victory. No one fell at the second fence, but at the third, the legend that was the late Tommy Carberry, four times Irish Champion National Hunt Jockey, came a cropper on L'Escargot. Tommy and the same horse had completed back-to-back Cheltenham Gold Cup victories in '70 and '71 and would go on to win the National in '75, preventing Red Rum from doing the straight treble. Tommy, the first jockey in history to win the Gold Cup, the Irish National and the English National, would even go on to train a Grand National winner piloted by his son, Paul, in 1999.

At the fourth, John Francome and Richard Pitman both fell. Just process those two names. Francome, Champion Jockey seven times, between 1976 and 1985, the third most successful National Hunt jump jockey of all time and Pitman, winner of the Champion

Hurdle, the King George twice, a Whitbread Gold Cup and a Hennessy Gold Cup. Yet, between the two of them, they were never destined to win one National, but boy was Richard Pitman going to go close the following year on the mighty Crisp. But that comes later.

For now, in the '72 running, Country Wedding and I were still on our feet. We continued to stay that way and I was absolutely chuffed to death when we cleared Becher's. That was such a thrill. We settled nicely for the next two fences, the Foinavon Fence and the Canal Turn and then it was Valentine's Brook. The ninth fence on the first circuit and one of the more famous. It's 5ft high and 3ft 3in wide with a brook on the landing side that's about 5ft 6in wide. The fence was originally known as the Second Brook, but was renamed after a horse named Valentine was reputed to have jumped the fence hind legs first in 1840. We didn't do anything half as fancy, we just ploughed through it and that was another National over for another year.

φ

Around the turn of the year I had started considering what I should be doing with my future. Now, as the season was drawing to a close, I knew it was coming to the crunch. It wasn't that I hadn't enjoyed working for Toby, I had and he had given me some fantastic opportunities, but the fact was, with only ten winners in the last year, I hadn't made any real progress. Yes, I was making a financial living, just about, but I wasn't making it into the top ranks of jockeys. I felt I was riding better than I had been, but the quality of the horses and the number of rides I was getting just weren't putting me into the mix. I knew it was time to consider my options.

Option one, to become the preferred jockey at Fyfield didn't seem likely. Eddie Harty had that position and there were much more experienced men lining up ahead of me. Option 2, stay put and keep trying, wasn't really an option either. Like I said before, Toby was a great man who, after racing was over for the day, was generous to a fault and kind, but the way he used to bollock me shattered my confidence. Option three was what was left; it was time to move on.

If I'm honest, I should have gone sooner. Maybe a year sooner, but I didn't and the final decision to move owes a lot to Eddie Harty and the sound advice he gave me, "You need to get out to become better."

I knew it was down to me having lost my claim too quickly and that Toby had lots of younger jockeys who still had their allowances, so I wasn't getting that many rides.

Eddie said it was quite straightforward, "You need to go Bobby. You can't just ride out around here and not for anybody else. Go and school some of Paul Cole's horses." Which I did.

Then I went on holiday to Cyprus in the summer break and on my return I moved in with Mary and her husband Richard on their farm just outside Wootton Bassett. I helped around the farm and tried to figure out how to secure rides for the new season. In the end it was simple. Mary and my then girlfriend went through the list of local racing stables and picked out the trainers that might need a jockey. One of the people they picked was Monty Stevens, who had recently bought Lucknam Park, near Chippenham and was converting it into a racing stable. I spoke to Monty's son, Jeffrey, rode out the following morning and within three days had been offered a retainer.

Monty, who sadly died in 1977, was a man of the country. He'd made his money as a farmer and cattle breeder and decided to start a racing stud. Then he started training his own horses, with no previous experience and enjoyed immediate success. He relied solely on instinct and I was told a long time later, that when he watched me that morning he apparently felt I was a natural. The other thing was that he wouldn't be on the track putting pressure on his jockeys. He preferred to sit in the comfort of his enormous living-room, listening to the betting-room commentaries.

Monty was a heck of a character. Yes, he loved his racehorses, but his true passion was racing pigeons. I remember I would go and have breakfast with him when I would be down there and on the morning of my first ride for him, I went to do the same. When I took my seat there wasn't much conversation so I mentioned that I'd seen a pigeon flying around and around outside in the yard. Monty got up and took a walk outside. After a while he came back in, lifted a twelve-bore shotgun, went back out, there was a bang and then Monty returned and took his seat at the table. As he picked his knife and fork up to continue with his breakfast he said casually, "That pigeon should have won. You'd better do the same this afternoon."

As a form of encouragement, I couldn't much argue with it. I did ask him a few days later why he'd got rid of the pigeon and he replied, "They're no damned good if they don't come back into the coup, they don't win races and they teach the others bad habits."

Thankfully my ride for him, on Winden at Devon and Exeter, ended with a twelve length victory. More winners followed. Other trainers began to reach out and hire me. I can see that the timing was quite fortunate because Jim Old, David Elsworth, who'd go on to train the magnificent Desert Orchid, and the late Patrick Haslam had all started training. Jim and David had been in Toby's the same as me, so we'd worked together before. Now they and Patrick were looking for me to ride for them. The decision to leave Toby was being vindicated.

φ

That October I had a strange old race at Wye. According to the official record, I won on a horse called Squiffy. But that never revealed the true story.

My Favourite Race
Apart from the obvious of Aldaniti in the National, I think my favourite race was at the lovely little course that was Wye. Nestled down in Kent, it was a 7-furlong loop that was tight in the extreme.

I was on Squiffy, a beautiful little mare with a neck no bigger than my arm, but who was simply nuts. She'd think nothing of trying to run away over the full length of a three mile chase. Although she and I had won a few together, so I felt I had the handling of her. This day we set off, jumped the first with no drama and then over the second my stirrup-leather broke. I couldn't pull her up if I'd wanted to, she was running away with me as usual, and there's not many I know who would take the decision to jump off a thoroughbred in full gallop, so I figured I'd kick my other stirrup out and stay with her. I remember thinking, 'She's small, I'll just keep on her for the last two and three-quarter miles 'bareback'. It'll not be easy, but it'll be fine.'

Now Wye was quite the rural setting and they'd shoo the sheep out of the weighing room and put an electric fence all around the inside of the track to stop them from straying onto the course.

On the first circuit, the jockey and later noted presenter and journalist Brough Scott, had fallen off, gone over the inside rail and got tangled up in the electric fence. So there's me riding bareback and there's Brough being slowly and not so quietly electrocuted by the sheep fence.

I think, for the three more circuits of Wye, it was the prospect of seeing Brough again, being contorted on the fence and twitching, which kept me on Squiffy. We didn't just keep going though, Squiffy put in her usual effort and with no brakes and not much in the way of steering, she was running away with it. She managed to negotiate each fence and by the last we were fifteen lengths clear, but I don't think I've laughed as much during a race before or since.

I'm glad to say Brough was fine. I know I won the grand total of £27 for that ride, but the amount of pain I had in my nether regions for the effort wasn't worth it. Although it might have been pay-back for laughing at Brough.

My first season as a freelancer was going okay and as the National approached I was asked by the trainer Desmond Dartnell if I would take the ride on a total outsider, Hurricane Rock. It had once been a useful chaser but had lost all its form since joining Dartnell's yard and although the SP was 100-1, if you had wanted to, you could have found bookies taking 500-1. But it was a ride in the National, so of course I was taking it.

Yet again I had no pressure on me and even if I had been at shorter odds, the pre-race expectation was all about the two top weights, L'Escargot and Crisp, and another little horse called Red Rum. Thirty-eight of us set off with Crisp and Red Rum starting as joint favourites.

By the time we got to Becher's on the first circuit, Crisp had started picking up speed and at the Canal Turn, he was out on his own in the lead.

I was tracking about ten or fifteen lengths back alongside Sunny Lad, who had my changing room neighbour, Bill Smith in the saddle. Crisp was pulling away with each stride.

Bill looked ahead and then shouted over to me, "He'll stop you know, he'll stop."

It didn't seem likely. As we approached the Chair, Crisp was at least twenty lengths clear of his nearest rival and just kept going further and further away. By the time we got to Becher's second time round, he was almost a full fence ahead of the rest of the field, apart from one. Red Rum, being ridden by the late, great Brian Fletcher had decided the time to mount a challenge had come.

So far Hurricane Rock had given me the most terrific ride and when Brian made his move, I did think to try to go with him, but we just weren't anywhere near good enough. However, Hurricane Rock did respond in his own way and so you can imagine my surprise when, turning into the home stretch, I found myself in third place on my 100-1 outsider.

If you watch the reruns, Crisp and Red Rum come round that last turn to the second last flight and I can just be seen on the outside of Spanish Steps and Rouge Autumn coming into the straight. We kept plugging along and held third place for a while, but eventually on that long, long run in, the brave Hurricane Rock was legless and almost stopped to a walk. Despite that, we finished sixth. It was the greatest, biggest thrill in racing I had ever had. I cannot tell you how chuffed I was at finishing. I had never known an emotion quite like it. More so because no one gave us a chance. Also, what a race to have my first National finish in.

I can always say, that yes, I was part of the 1973 classic that saw the gallant, heart-breaking effort by Dick Pitman on Crisp, the class act Australian chaser, who was not just top weight, but was carrying twenty-three pounds more than the rival who was closing in on him with every stride. It's no wonder that the '73 run-in features in many a person's favourite sporting moments. Crisp, having led by so much and for so long, was past the Elbow and heading to the finish line but tying up with each yard. Behind him, the little battler who would go on to be a legend. Even in the final furlong it didn't look possible, but in the last five strides Red Rum closed the gap and won by three-quarters of a length. What a race!

As I turned Hurricane Rock towards the unsaddling enclosure, Bill Smith crossed the line on Sunny Lad in fifteenth place. I raised my whip in acknowledgement and shouted over, "You were right Bill, he did stop, but it took a bloody long time!"

A lot of people have given their opinions about Crisp and Richard Pitman's tactics that day. Personally I think he was by far the best horse never to have won the race and was simply beaten by three things.

The trip, the weight and Red Rum.

Bill Smith was a great character and like all of us, had to be able to take a joke. At Windsor one year he was given the ride on one of Her Majesty Queen Elizabeth, the Queen Mother's horses. I loved the Queen Mother; she was a genuine lady, knew her racehorses and had a great affection and affinity for jump racing. I can't think that we've ever had a better supporter of National Hunt racing than she and it always makes me smile nowadays when I see the magnificent bronze bust of her at the side of the Parade Ring in Cheltenham. It captures her spirit beautifully and is a fitting tribute to a wonderful person.

But, back on that day at Windsor, Bill had come out to get mounted up without realising someone had tacked a pair of red tights onto the back of his colours. He should have been stopped before he got to the ring, but had slipped through and then we were all caught out by the fact the Queen Mum was coming up to him. It was too late and we all held our breath. We needn't have worried. Her

Majesty took a quick look at the red tights dangling from his backside and said, "I'd rather you didn't wear those today. They'll clash terribly with one's colours."

I ended my first 'freelance' season with a better than one-in-ten win return. Twenty-nine wins from 227 rides. I knew the decision to leave Toby's had been the correct one.

One of the more unusual of those twenty-nine winners had been as the season was drawing to a close. As I've said before, I'm not a drinker. Maybe it was seeing Dad drink or that night with the young jockeys, either way I never really over indulged, however the night of the 'Horse & Hounds' Ball in the spring of 1973 was a real exception! I blame Derek as he was with me and I only made it home at 7am the following morning with a blinding hangover.

I just about managed to get to Stratford where I was meant to be riding a horse called Unavailable for 'Frenchy' Nicholson and his son David, 'The Duke', who took one look at me and said, "If I were you Bob, I'd have a couple of brandies or you're fit for nothing!"

Now no one had ever won on this horse so expectations weren't high. I did as advised and gave that horse the best ride of its life and we won. To be honest I don't really remember the race and had I been sober I'm not sure we'd have won! It's the only time I've ever been in that state, but it was one of the best races of my career!

And no, I don't think you'd get away with it now!

φ

The new season started fantastically for me. I even led the Jockey's Championship for a few weeks. It was great! It got even better when Josh Gifford came calling.

He was looking for a new stable jockey as sadly his previous one, Doug Barrott, had been fatally injured at Newcastle on April the 28th whilst riding French Colonist in the Whitbread Gold Cup. As the horse fell, Doug's foot had become trapped in the stirrup and he was dragged for a considerable distance. He died on May the 3rd 1973, at the age of just twenty-six. Doug had been the seventh jockey to die in a race in the previous seven years. Death and injury on the track is something that you almost come to expect, but it doesn't make it easier when we lose one of our colleagues and friends.

By the August, Josh had whittled his choices for a replacement down to me or Richard Evans and decided that he'd give us both chances on his horses. Basically, whoever did best would get the job. Sadly my first outing for him, at Kempton in a three-horse novice chase, ended up with me being dumped off the 16-1 outsider, Clare Dawn. Josh ran over to me, checked I was okay, then helped me remount and I managed to finish and claim the third place prize money. It wasn't the most auspicious start, but Josh offered me a few more rides and thankfully I started giving him winners. Before too long he offered me a retainer for the season. It was a fantastic opportunity yet mixed with sadness at taking over in poor Doug Barrott's spot. I suppose it was walking in dead man's shoes. Of course I took it, but I still felt funny about it.

Josh Gifford was one of the best trainers in the country and a former four times Champion Jockey. Never having been a faller in all his rides around Aintree, he was the man who, on Honey End, had finished second to Foinavon in that famous 1967 National. He was also a true gentleman, someone who would become my friend and someone who, in a few years, would be pivotal to my survival. But that was for the future. In 1973 he chose me to ride because, in an interview he gave later, he said,

"The best jockey is the one who has the fewest falls and it was clear Bob was a superb horseman. Jumping is the name of the game. If horses jump then they are going to win races. A race is won from the time the starting gate goes up, out in the country, by a sympathetic rider who gets them round in the most economical way. Also Bob was not a man who resorted to the whip very often. I'm against whip jockeys.

A jockey who rides with a sensible length of stirrup doesn't have to use the stick too much. Remember if a

horse doesn't go for one or two cracks, he's not going to go for twelve."

The 73-74 season was the start of a fantastic few years when Josh and I had a great run of success. I was achieving what I'd always wanted to, but alongside the ups, were the constant downs as I continued to battle my weight issues.

I can admit now that I tried all manner of 'remedies', some less than wise, in the effort to keep my weight low. The saunas and the Turkish Baths in Gloucester, which I'd share with John Haine and Terry Biddlecombe, were the more social, fun and I suppose, normal activities. The 'Piss Pills' I've already mentioned, in conjunction with taking laxatives, were on the more extreme side. Finally, on one occasion, I decided to try a more severe method. There was a doctor in London who would inject a powerful diuretic that caused dehydration and led to a brief, but rapid drop in weight. You followed the injection up with some pills that contained a stimulant which speeded up the system and dulled your appetite. I drove myself down to his practice and he injected me in the backside and the pain of it was staggering, literally. Then he gave me two boxes of pills, spoke to me for a bit and then showed me out. I could barely hobble and after a short distance I passed out in the street. Thankfully a passing traffic warden helped me back to my car and for the next two hours I sat in the driver's seat sweating buckets. It was the first and only time in London that I hadn't had to worry about getting a parking ticket!

I made it home eventually, but the pills made me so ill I stopped taking them long before I made it through even the first box. However, I'm not too sure John Francome's recollections of me are accurate, because I couldn't believe what he sent me for inclusion into this book.

"Bob Champion, my favourite memory of him? That's easy.

He'd walk in to the weighing room and have a cuppa and two sandwiches. You'd ask him how his weight was going and he'd say, 'Oh it's terrible, I haven't eaten in twenty-four hours' and he'd still have crumbs round his mouth. He'd swear blind he hadn't eaten. It was a standing joke that if you wanted a sarnie you had to get in the weighing room before Bob. He had food amnesia. He'd forget he'd eaten as soon as he swallowed it."

I'm sure he's got me confused with someone else!

I didn't get offered a ride in the '74 National, but as the season drew to a close I overcame that disappointment by going on holiday to Minorca with a whole gaggle of other jockeys and their wives, including my mate Bob Davies. The married men didn't seem to be having as good a time as I was, but I couldn't let that stop me from enjoying the sun and the sea, the nightclubs, the partying and the occasional companions I would meet.

During the day all the jockeys would go swimming, hire boats and try out at water skiing. Being a competitive bunch each would strive to be the best in endurance tests. I have to confess that Bob was not only a better jockey than me, he was a much better water skier.

φ

I returned to Josh's yard after the break, raring to go and sure enough, I had my best season to date. I was in the top six of the Jockey Championship again and really felt that I was beginning to properly make my mark. With no ride in the '74 National I was keen not be left out again and so I was delighted when in the '75 running, I was back in a field of thirty-one on board the 40-1 outsider Manicou Bay. This was the year Red Rum, under Brian Fletcher, was aiming for a third straight success but who was giving away 11lbs to the mighty L'Escargot under Tommy Carberry. It was a difference that was just too much and L'Escargot won by fifteen lengths, thereby emulating Golden Miller's achievement of being a Cheltenham Gold Cup and Aintree Grand National winner, albeit not in the same year. Even now, they're still the only two steeplechase horses ever to have achieved that remarkable feat.

As for me and Manicou Bay, we'd had a lovely clear run round. Travelling just behind L'Escargot for the majority of a brutal first circuit that had seen the field reduced to just sixteen, I then tucked in behind Red Rum until he accelerated away. I dropped in behind L'Escargot again and although eventually left by the pace of both of them, I nevertheless managed, for the second time in my career, to get up to finish sixth.

I was thrilled and the race had been as exciting as ever, but one of the things I remember is the strangest unseating of a rider I think I'd ever seen. Andy Turnell on April Seventh, was literally flung up, forward and to the left after his horse landed heavily at Becher's first time round. As he was in mid-air he put his hand out to stop himself from crashing into the jockey next to him, Paul Kelleway on Barona. All he actually managed to do was grab Kelleway's arm and pull him out of the saddle. Both jockeys ended up on the turf. Paul was not a happy chap, yet any animosity between the two was instantly forgotten as they went to the aid of Spittin' Image's jockey who was lying prone just behind them. Thankfully he was alright after a spot of time with the medics.

It's indicative of how we jockeys used to band together. We were our own particular 'club' and felt a great affinity for one another. Richard Pitman tells a funny story. He was having breakfast with Fred Winter, a stern but really lovely man, prior to riding for him that day. As they were chatting Fred told his wife, Di, that I was taking their daughter, Denise, out. Well Di got very quiet for a moment and then said, with a little reproof to her voice, "But Fred, he's only a jockey isn't he?"

Fred looked at her and said quite seriously, "Well darling, what was I?"

I guess that gave me the green light. I dread to think what would have happened had Fred not been okay with it!

The season ended well and the new one started just as brightly. The winners kept coming and I was loving life. On the 25th October, at the Cambridgeshire track of Huntingdon, notably the town where Josh had been born, I rode four of his horses to victory on the one day, my best ever. I was by now knocking on the door of the Jockey Championship's top three and was financially much more secure.

I've lived in a great many places over the years, some more fancy than others. I shared rooms as a young jockey and then progressed to sharing houses, like Mrs Atherton's thatched cottage where I lived with Robin Barwell, Jim Old and Gardie Grissell, but I'll never forget the thrill of owning my first home.

I became the proud owner of a small house in Shelbourne. I thought it was a palace and I lived there for five years. If I'm honest, it's probably my favourite home of all the ones I've had because it was the first that was all mine. It seemed like I was a proper grown-up.

I was terribly house proud, would often have dinner parties and was, I am slightly embarrassed to say, known for plumping cushions as soon as a visitor stood up and for clearing and washing up between courses. I think I took being house proud to extreme levels sometimes, but it was a novelty and I loved being tidy. I still do, but not quite to those extremes. I just like things being in their proper places and everything kept neat.

In the '76 running of the National I was on the 2nd shortest priced horse I would ever ride in the race. Trained by the ever colourful Verley Bewicke and going off at 12-1, the joint third favourite, behind Red Rum and Barona, Money Market was in the form of his life. He had won a second consecutive Peter Cazalet/Mildmay Memorial at Sandown and in the Cheltenham Gold Cup had made most of the running before fading to finish fourth. Confirming his form, we contested the lead, and led for long stretches, right from the off until crossing the Melling Road for the second time. As we headed back out into the country I could feel him slacken and we went from first to seventh in what felt like a few strides. After a bit of a melee at Becher's, we were dropped right off the leading group and I knew my job was just to keep him going and see the race out. We finished 14th but it was another finish and had allowed me to lead a National for the better part of a circuit. It was all valuable experience that I hoped I could build on as each year went by.

The next opportunity, in 1977, was going to be tougher as I was on the very experienced, but 50-1 outsider, Spittin' Image. Forty-two runners lined up for what was to become the most famous of all the modern Grand Nationals; Red Rum's historic third victory. Not widely known is that his jockey for that day, Tommy Stack, was offered a live mic hook-up by the BBC to record his audio on the race, but he changed his mind in the weighing room when he saw the fairly bulky equipment and in the end the mic was carried by Graham Thorner instead. Graham forgot about it and subsequently none of the recording could be used as he mostly swore for the three minutes he was on board Prince Rock and swore a lot more when he fell off at the 12th.

As for me, well, I got to watch the fantastic Red Rum win because my race ended, with six others, at a mass pile up at the very first fence. It was a huge anti-climax after the previous few years.

ϕ

The day before that National I'd had a win at Ascot on a horse that I'd ridden for the first time in 1975. It had been foaled in 1970 at the Harrogate Stud in Darlington to a mostly mediocre breeding line. Subsequently, we would learn that he shared the same fifth dam as Grundy, the eventual 1975 Derby winner, but that race hadn't been run as yet when he was sold for 3,200 guineas to Josh Gifford at the Ascot Bloodstock Sales in May 1974. Josh ran him for the first time on 10th January 1975 at Ascot and I had the ride. It was the Silver Doctor Novices' Hurdle (Div 2) and we had gone off at a starting price of 33-1 carrying 11st. I recall it was a big field of seventeen and one of them, Sunnyboy, owned by the Queen Mother, was expected to win easily. Instead I romped home by four lengths, surprising quite a few people. There was something immediately apparent in this headstrong horse. I liked him straight away.

One of Josh's owners, Nick Embiricos, also liked him and had asked if he could be given first refusal if Josh thought about selling him. Josh, ever the business man, sold him to Nick shortly after that maiden win for a reasonable profit. Sadly though, the horse wouldn't win over hurdles again because he suffered a serious strain to the tendon on his right foreleg. It took thirteen months, a bar firing operation and a long rest in the Barkford Manor Stud before he could come back on to the track. When he did, he was switched to steeplechasing. Josh, myself, Nick and his wife Valda all felt he'd do better with the bigger fences. So it was, after the long layoff that I joined up with him again at Newbury. He unseated me on that first return, but then the day before the '77 Grand National, we won. It was a good feeling to be back on-board one of the country's most promising chasers. I also liked the fact he'd been named for the four grandchildren of his breeder, Tommy Barron, with the first two letters from Alastair, David, Nicola and Timothy being put together to form Aldaniti.

In early November we won the Silver Fox Chase at Leicester and when I came back into the winner's enclosure I said to Josh, Nick and Valda, "That horse will win the National one day." It wasn't a glib statement. I was sure of it. I instinctively knew it. You may wonder just how I knew it, but I'd been fortunate in my career to have ridden horses before they went off and actually won the National. I've already told you about winning on Highland Wedding in the race before he won at Aintree in '69. I'd won on Rag Trade in his very first race over fences and he'd go on to win the big one in '76. I also used to look after Rubstic, the '79 winner, when he was a two year old, so I knew what a National horse was like. From day one I knew that Aldaniti was a National horse and the Leicester victory just sealed it for me.

Sometimes you need to pay attention to the convictions and feelings that you have. A few years' later it proved crucial that the owners had indeed paid attention.

At the end of November, Aldaniti repaid my conviction in him with giving me my best ride in a big race to date. We lined up at Newbury for the Hennessy Cognac Gold Cup (now the Ladbrokes Trophy). Originally handicapped for 10st dead, Josh and Nick knew there was no way I'd make that weight, so they said I'd still have the ride if I could make 10st 7lb, which I did. The Hennessy is 3miles 2½furlongs and is prestigious due to some of the horses that have won it as a precursor to even greater things. In the 1960s, Millhouse and Arkle (twice) won it and it continues to be a superb indicator for the following year's Cheltenham Gold Cup with it most recently revealing the likes of Denman and Bob's Worth.

In the 1977 running we set off quite well, but Aldaniti went straight through the 2nd fence and it practically stopped us dead. When he'd regained his balance we were in pursuit of a field that was now about twenty lengths distant. It's a testament to him that by the second last we were back in contention, but the catching up had taken the wind out of him and the best we could hang on for was a credible third.

It was this race that I got into trouble with the Jockey Club for having been weighed in 4lbs heavier than I'd weighed out. The stewards demanded to know what the reason was and I swore that all I'd had between weighing out and in was a cup of tea. I think it would all have gone away if the press hadn't got hold of the story and blown it out of proportion. So it was that the Jockey Club had to be seen to carry out a thorough investigation for which I was thankfully cleared of all blame.

Given his performance, it was possible Aldaniti might have been set for a tilt at the Cheltenham Gold Cup the following year, but sadly it was soon apparent that he'd gone lame. In fact he had chipped two pieces of bone off his pastern, just below his fetlock on his off-hind (right-hind) leg. It was assessed that he'd done it with the almighty blunder at that 2nd fence and yet he'd continued for three miles and finished in the frame. He was one tough horse.

The vets determined that the only hope of him ever racing again was a period of complete rest. Again he went back to Barkford and was restricted to his box from December 1977 through to July 1978. That is an incredibly long time for a thoroughbred racehorse to be cooped up and for him to come through it owed so much to Head Girl, Beryl Millem, along with her two assistants Lin Wilcox and Margaret Phillips. It was quite amazing that when Aldaniti was led out of his box in July, he was fully recovered.

Whilst Aldaniti was out of action, I continued riding for Josh with a fair amount of success, although at Cheltenham that December I suffered the worst fall of my career. It's truly the only time I thought I was going to die on a racecourse. It was in a novice chase and I was on a horse called Billet Doux II. We clipped the top of one of the fences going down the hill on the far side of the track and the horse flipped me into the ground. He brought down another runner who did a double-somersault and landed straight on top of me. Every last bit of breath was crushed out of me and the pain was so much worse than anything I'd ever felt. I know it sounds like a cliché, but yes, I genuinely did see my life pass before me. It was in slow motion and seemed to take for ages, both the bad and the good were all there in front of me. I was obviously knocked out and when I came round I still couldn't breathe. I went out again and dreamt that I was dead. But whoever decides these things didn't want me at that time, so I woke up in the ambulance with an oxygen mask on my face. I was incredibly lucky that the course doctor had been travelling close behind the on-track ambulance and luckier still to come away with only a broken shoulder and some damaged ribs. I was taken off to hospital but, as usual, discharged myself and went home. I managed to have a bit of a sleep, had a bath in the morning but struggled to get back out of it. I went to London to see Doctor Alun Thomas, the go-to doctor for all of us jump jockeys. He sorted me out although I was literally black and blue. I couldn't ride again for ten days. It was during that break that I remembered about the whole life passing in front of my eyes moment. I was quite shocked by it but also quite buoyed that I hadn't had any horrendous feelings of regret. It just was what it was. After the ten days my strong season continued, even though I kept missing out on a lot of rides due to my weight issues.

Back at Aintree the following April, I was on board the 16-1 shot Shifting Gold and when Tied Cottage, owned by a man I much admired, Anthony Robinson, went at Becher's first time round, I found myself in the lead next to Lucius and Double Bridle. That lasted until Valentine's when we made a hash of it and the horse became totally unsettled. I managed to keep going to the next when he just folded underneath me. Another year gone, but at least my old mate Bob Davies went on to win on Lucius.

I couldn't even be that disappointed, because I finished that season with the best total I ever managed. I was third in the Jockey's Championship with 56 winners, and when you see that first was Jonjo O'Neill and second was John Francombe, I can't be too displeased at all. Josh also returned his best total as a trainer to date with 82 winners. We were thriving.

Added to our success was the stable's American amateur jockey, George Sloan. He'd quite remarkably become the British Amateur Jockey Champion with a total of 23 wins. It was a great victory of good old fashioned planning. George, who owned a myriad of health spas in Tennessee, trained his own horses and hosted the annual Hillsboro' Foxhounds on his fourteen hundred acre estate near Nashville, had teamed up with a bunch of friends to found the Tennessee Jubilee Sports Syndicate. They'd gone off and purchased a string of horses, put most of them with Josh and at the end of the year got the majority of their investment back by selling them on. The profit, and I believe a substantial one, was made from backing at very, very lucrative odds, George to win the Amateur Championship.

George and I got on well, so when he invited me to go over to the States for the summer, I didn't hesitate. My idea was to start riding out for some local trainers and maybe establish myself in the US, but jump racing is a very poor cousin to the flat over there and the number of rides are limited. Although the prize money was far and away better than the UK, so it made up for it.

I started working for Jonathan Sheppard, an English trainer doing well there and I stayed for a while with an American jockey, Tommy Skiffington, who I'd known when he was riding in England a few years earlier. It wasn't that long before Burly Cocks, a veteran trainer out of Unionville, Pennsylvania asked me to ride for him in a race at Delaware. I finished fourth but Burly had liked what he'd seen and I ended the week riding in four jump races and giving Tommy Voss, another noted trainer, a winner on Wild Sir. The thing I remember most about it was the common changing rooms with the flat jockeys. That's how I came to meet the likes of Angel Cordero, the legendary Willie Shoemaker and a young up and coming jockey nicknamed, 'The Kid'; Steve Cauthen.

I was able to stay for a bit longer than normal as Josh told me that because the tracks back home were so firm he wouldn't be running any of his horses until later in the season. I ended up in Saratoga riding for Tommy Voss again and won three more races on

Wild Sir. It was such a great experience and I think I fell in love with the US a little. Then I headed back to England to be Josh Gifford's first choice jockey.

φ

In November '78 it was back to Newbury and another tilt at the Hennessey, but this time on Approaching. Yet again it was only Josh and the owner, Major Derek Wigan, who had faith enough in me to post four pounds over the handicapped weight of 10st 2lb. Even then, for me to get to 10st 6lb was an effort. I starved and sweated for five days and recall emerging from the Newbury changing-room grey faced, haggard and freezing. I had to pull on an overcoat. Seriously, I was freezing and I knew it was down to all the fasting and wasting. Thankfully no one ever asked me to make that weight again.

> *Major Wigan was a very enthusiastic owner and he loved to bet, more importantly to win. He and I had a great relationship and when it came to the Hennessy Gold Cup he made it known he REALLY wanted a win. I was already fasting to reach what seemed an impossible target and not in a great mood. I saw Major Wigan the day before the big race and he asked what I was on that afternoon. When I told him what I was riding in a novice chase he immediately knew that this horse wouldn't be a winner and would in fact likely fall and possibly injure the rider. He looked straight at me and said, "That horse'll bury you, you won't be riding."*
>
> *It's the first and only time an owner pulled me from a race I'd been booked to ride, but I'm so glad he did. I can't actually remember the horse's name now but I do know that it indeed buried the jockey and injured him badly. Had it been me I wouldn't have been fit to ride in the Hennessy.*

But, I had made it and so I set off on Approaching amidst a field of eight.

I was fairly confident, because Approaching was a four times course winner at Newbury and so he knew his way around it. I took him onto the inside, next to Orillo and sat tight on what I knew was a real unorthodox jumper. He never seemed to flex his back the way most steeplechasers do, but he made up for it by being big, yet nimble. Whichever way he jumped, it worked and more often than not he made his way over obstacles. So it was that we hit the front six out and I decided to give him his head. He was flying and five out we went two lengths clear of William Pen, with Orillo in third. Approaching accelerated again and at the fourth last we had four or five lengths in hand. Behind me, Orillo and then William Pen were being reeled in by the fast improving Master H. By the third last, Master H was clear in second and closing in on us, but he stumbled on landing, handing us a clear advantage. We cleared the second last with ease, while Master H lumbered over it. William Pen, a long way behind in third was not going to be a danger.

At the final fence, it seemed that all of my fasting and wasting and freezing had been worthwhile, for Approaching rewarded me with an outstanding leap, standing off and gaining lengths in the air. The only opposition, Master H, never got closer than five lengths. It was comfortable. I'd just won the Hennessey Gold Cup!

The celebrations were, umm robust, might be the best word. I had a prawn cocktail, (ah how that dates it), steak, salad, two helpings of ice cream and copious glasses of champagne. The following day I found that I had put on ten pounds.

On Boxing Day, I travelled to Kempton for the King George VI Chase meeting but I wasn't riding in the Chase, rather I'd be on Kybo in the prestigious Christmas Hurdle, a Grade One race and part of hurdling's 'Triple Crown'. It meant that my Christmas dinner had been severely curtailed and there hadn't been much in the way of mince pies, but it was worth it as Kybo, an outstanding hurdler and one of the best horses I ever rode, came home for the victory. I wondered if this season could get better. It did indeed, although it nearly became amazing.

After the Christmas success we took Kybo to Cheltenham for the biggest prize in hurdling, the Champion Hurdle. There was a little bit of pressure as the press felt that Kybo would win. In my gut I didn't think he would. Racing down the hill, approaching the second last, we had the superb Monksfield and Sea Pigeon in attendance, but we weren't just going with those two legends, we were holding them easily. I began to wonder if we might not have this in the bag after all and I was still thinking that when we clattered the hurdle and slithered to the ground. I was so fed up I sat on the turf for a good couple of minutes. I know there was still a distance to go and I know that those two prolific horses had a tremendous battle to the line, but honestly, in the heat of the moment I reckoned Kybo and I would have beaten them... but in my heart, with the distance of time, I don't really think we would have. Ah, we'll never really know. Although our not winning did at least prove my gut instincts right and they were confirmed again when we ran second to Monksfield a few weeks later. Mind you, there was no shame in running second to a horse like Monksfield.

I should probably add in here that whereas the Aintree Grand National is by far the biggest and most famous race in the National Hunt calendar, it is the Cheltenham Festival, held during March, that is the most prestigious meeting in the sport and home to not only the Champion Hurdle but also the richest non-handicap chase in Britain, often referred to as the Blue Riband of National Hunt Racing; the Cheltenham Gold Cup.

I've said already that the Hennessey Gold Cup was a good indicator for the following year's Cheltenham Gold Cup, so Josh was determined we would set up for it, but cruelly, Approaching had been injured soon after his Newbury triumph. Instead, we would fall back on a returning old friend; Aldaniti.

So it was, that on Thursday, 15th March 1979, Aldaniti and I, at a starting price of 40-1, rode into the teeth of a 'Cheltenham Spring' snowstorm.

I held off quite near the rear and tracked a strung out field following Anthony Robertson's Tied Cottage with the magnificent Tommy Carberry, a three-time Gold Cup winner, on board. By the time we got to the second fence, Tied Cottage was already an incredible ten lengths clear. We set off out into the country and at the crown of the hill I found myself next to the imperious hurdler, Night Nurse, with my good mate Ian Watkinson in the saddle. I looked across to my left and the snow was that thick you could hardly see the grandstands on the other side of the course. The conditions were brutal. We completed the first circuit, slogged up the hill and back out into the country for the second time with Tied Cottage now twenty lengths distant from Royal Mail and Alverton.

I had been detached from the main following group of six horses and you could have been forgiven for thinking the winner and minor places would be coming from the far off leader and that group, but Aldaniti wasn't done just yet. Descending the hill second time round, Night Nurse started falling off the pace and I picked up my rhythm, but I was still a long, long way from the business end of the race.

As the leaders cleared the fourth last, Alverton and Royal Mail were reeling in Tied Cottage, and the prescient master of commentators, Peter O'Sullevan, said, "And these three, bar a fall, have the 1979 Gold Cup between them."

Alverton, with Jonjo O'Neill on board, was pressing the long-time leader hard, but Carberry held steady. In what was becoming a classic, the two were stride for stride and neck and neck at the last flight but Tied Cottage, tired from his exertions, went right through the top of it and his forelegs folded under him. The collective sigh from the grandstand was something to hear. The thing about race goers, be they owners, trainers or punters, is that they all love a brave, honest trier and Tied Cottage was the epitome of that.

Jonjo was left twenty five lengths clear and rode Alverton hands and heels up the famous Cheltenham Hill to victory. Royal Mail so nearly came a cropper at the last but held on and I found myself, twenty lengths further behind, in a tussle with Casamayor. We cleared the last and honestly, I was amazed by the tremendous way Aldaniti rallied. We stormed up the hill and took third in a photo finish. I was truly delighted. Third in the Cheltenham Gold Cup!

The Irish always send their best to Cheltenham, both the horses and the jockeys. Some of those Irish lads can be quite big fellas and you'd definitely want them on your side if anyone was ever giving you any grief in the town of an evening. Because of the size of them, they'd always join the rest of us 'poor souls' in some hard fasting and wasting in the saunas of Cheltenham each morning before the racing started. When I say hard wasting, I mean it. You probably haven't eaten properly in a week and your body is in partial shutdown. It's not the greatest feeling in the world.

One day, Steve Smith-Eccles, who was a slightly made chap and annoyingly never needed to worry about his weight, decided to live up to his reputation as the liveliest, funniest and most outrageous prankster in the changing room. I will grant him that, he was a funny bugger. This particular day he thought it would be hilarious to wander into the sauna with a great big hotdog, dripping with to-mato sauce and mustard and offer everyone a bite.

It didn't take many seconds for him to figure out he had gone a bit too far with the Irish boys. He just about made it out and away before they caught him, or otherwise I'm not too sure where that hotdog would have ended up.

The season, by far my most successful, if not in winning numbers, had bounded along and I found myself back at Aintree on the New Zealand horse, Purdo. A 25-1 shot, but starting price is no indicator of National glory and I was flattered by him as we led on the inside for the first five fences. He was jumping like a star and I began to wonder if this was going to be my year. I was still contemplating it when I approached the mighty Becher's clear and going easy. He half corkscrewed over it, put his front legs through it and was completely outdone by the drop on the other side. As he crumpled onto the ground I was flung clear, ended up sitting on my backside and was then run over by one of the others. A typical day in a National Hunt jockey's life really, resulting in just the usual bruises and wounded pride.

Shortly after the race I noticed small lumps under my nipples. I went to see Dr Alun Thomas in Park Lane. He advised me simply to lose weight by sweating in the saunas. I went and sweated and sure enough, they went away. All was good. I let the doctor know. He told me that was indeed good, but to see him urgently should they return.

A few weeks later I was due to ride in the Scottish Grand National, but the day before it I went to the flat races in Newbury. I liked watching the flat races and often rode out for Paul Cole. My Mum had asked me to have a bet for her and so I put a £10 accumulator on five horses. The first four won and Mum had about £9,000 going on to the last. Not that she knew about it just yet! My selection for her in the fifth was a 3-1 shot and the jockey was a good young apprentice of Paul's called Mark Malham. I thought we had it in the bag, but Mark dropped his stick at the furlong marker and got beat a short head. It cost my mother in the region of £36,000! I decided not to tell her.

I got in my car and readied myself to take the long drive to Scotland. I was hoping to have some very attractive female company, in fact, I thought it was a sure thing, but alas my would-be date bailed on me. I remember thinking, 'Uh oh, bad luck comes in threes.'

Aldaniti and I met up at Ayr and we were all set. At 4miles and 110yards the Scottish Grand National is only 400yards shorter than the Aintree edition and is a fair test of a steeplechaser. There's not many have managed to do a Scottish-English double and only one horse has ever won both in the same year, but of course, what else would you have expected from Red Rum?

In the April '79 running, we went off as the 9-2 favourite. After a couple of circuits, we were travelling nicely in second or third and had wound in the early long-distance leader, Flashy Boy. As the pace began to increase we came to the first of the five fences on the far side of the course and a huge mistake from Flashy Boy saw Aldaniti and me take the lead. We were travelling so well and I thought, with more than half a circuit to go, I should hold him, make sure he didn't run out of steam, so I pulled back and let the field close up. As we made the homeward turn I began to release him a bit and we eased back into the lead by a length from Royal Stuart. We took the third last still about a length to the good and I thought we stood a really good chance of taking the race, but Fairview, ridden by Ridley Lamb, was rallying hard. We took the second last stride for stride, but on the level ground Aldaniti had a speed advantage and once more pulled about a length clear going to the final fence.

Halfway to it, I could feel him beginning to struggle, but I squeezed him tight and waved my whip hand a couple of times. He responded and put us another length to the good over Fairview and I heard a great cheer rising in the crowd. I settled Aldaniti, straightened him up, gave him a kick and got a good jump out of him over the last. I pulled into the middle of the course, Fairview went to the rails and then, as if from nowhere, the local Scottish hope, Fighting Fit, with Colin Hawkins on board was almost level with me on the outside. That was what the crowd were cheering.

It was all down to what speed we had left over the run in. I urged Aldaniti on and we kept up our gallop, but Fighting Fit closed us down with every stride. At the fifty yard mark we were nose for nose. I gave Aldaniti a reminder but saw that Colin had only given Fighting Fit a quick slap to the neck and the horse passed us like we'd stopped. There was no way we were going to catch him, but I kept my concentration and we easily held on for second by 2½ lengths. Second in the Scottish Grand National!

The year just kept getting better and better. Well, apart from that third bit of bad luck I'd been waiting on. I'd told my Mum to bet on me and all four of my rides came in second that day at Ayr. Poor Mum hadn't taken them each-way so lost out again. I did get a nice comment from Josh though, a man of not many words, who said, "Don't feel bad Bob, you did everything right. You haven't deserved to come second best this afternoon." I'm often asked to give a tip on racing and my advice to anyone is always the same now, "You want a tip? Don't bet on horses! Keep your money in your pocket! Even a sure thing can lose on the day."

Despite those three strikes, the year had been tremendous. I started to think about the following season. How could I improve even more? How good could it be? I reckoned, with a little more effort and a touch of luck there was no reason to think it couldn't be really terrific. Basically, all I wanted to do was build on this season. I mean, I had a Hennessey, a Christmas Hurdle, a close run thing in the Champion Hurdle, a 3rd in the Gold Cup, 2nd in the Scottish Grand National and I lay 3rd in the Jockey Championship. Maybe next season I could take all of them up a step, or two. Maybe in '79-80 Aldaniti and I could go after the big one. Maybe next season… anything was possible.

I felt on top of the world.

I had no idea that in the early months of that next season, Aldaniti would be injured to the point of the vet recommending that he be euthanised, my career would have come to a sudden, terrible stop and that I'd be, quite literally, fighting for my life.

Image Set A:

1. Mum & Dad's Wedding 1946
2. With Dad at the Eridge Hunt
3. With Dad, Mary and the Cleveland Hounds
4. Alongside my great riding tutor, Margaret Neesham
5. A dressed up photo with Dad and Mary
6. Roseberry Topping, Yorkshire, where Mum & Dad's ashes are scattered
7. Mounted on my pony Pinto
8. Me turning hay
9. My first winner. Holmcourt, in the Tedworth Adjacent Hunts, Larkhill, March 1964.
10. Training in the States as I recovered
11. With Josh and Aldaniti in the yard at Findon
12. First winner for Josh Gifford on Captain Hardy at Windsor
13. With Mary and little Nick
14. My first winner, Wild Sir, in America
15. With Carol the Ward Sister at the Royal Marsden
16. Golden Spurs Winners (Me next to the great Lester Piggott and sporting quite the black eye).
17. The Guv'nor Josh Gifford
18. The great Burly Cocks
19. Me doing my best Mr Darcy impression in Japan
20. My old riding peg in the Aintree Racecourse changing room
21. Speaking to Her Majesty the Queen Mother after my first runner for her, which finished 4th at Newbury

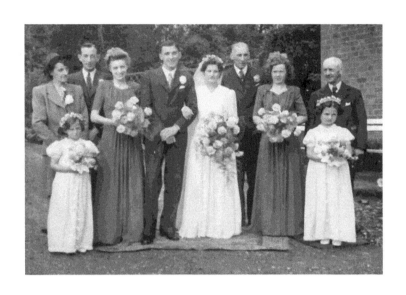

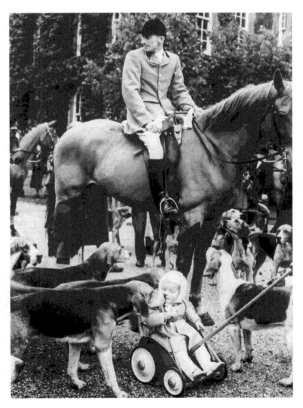

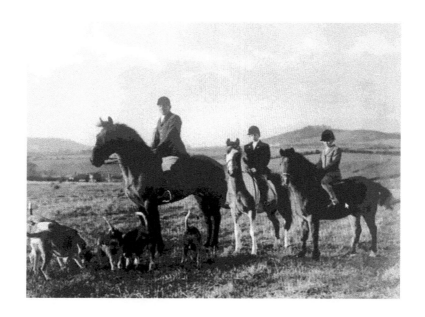

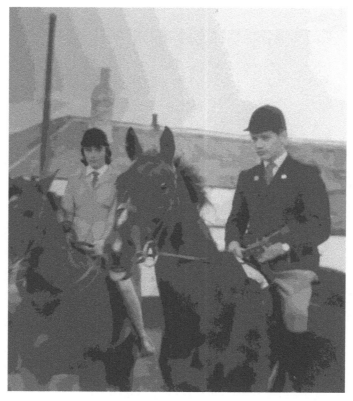

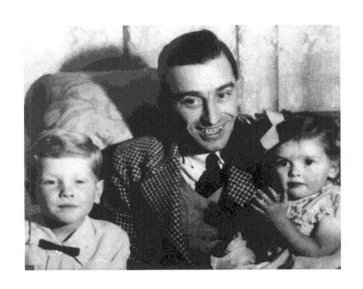

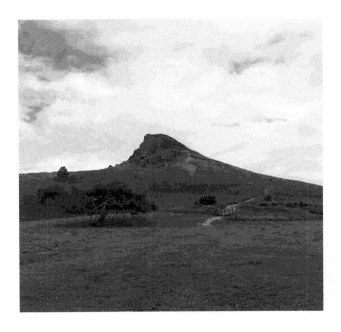

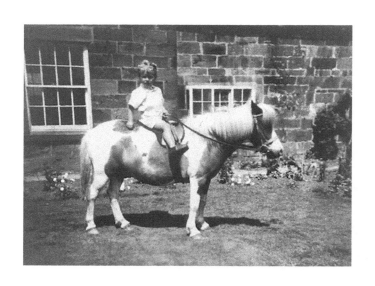

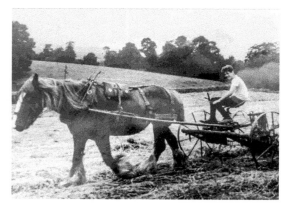

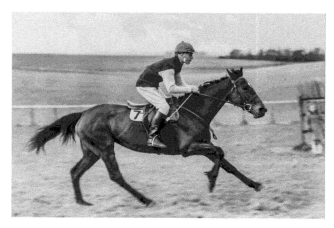

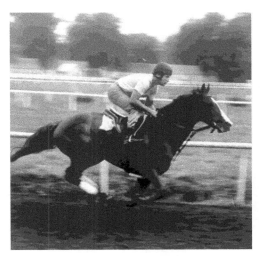

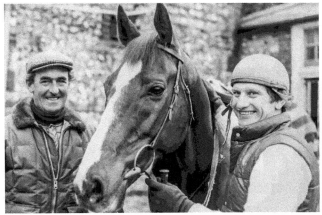

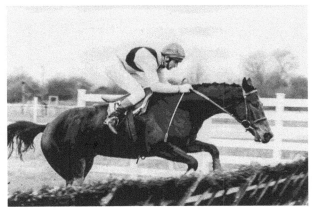

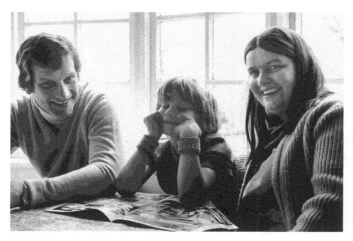

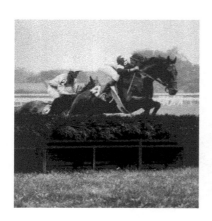

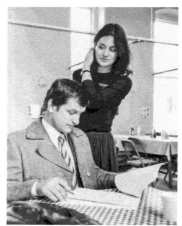

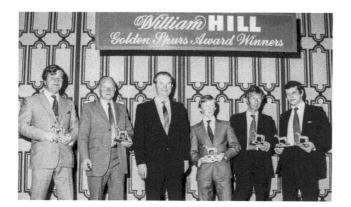

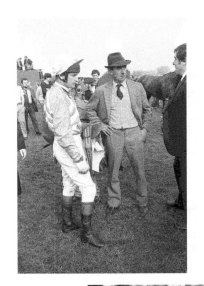
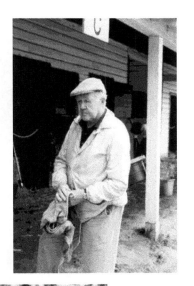
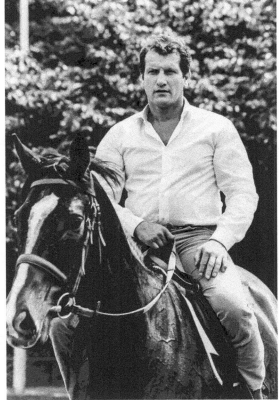

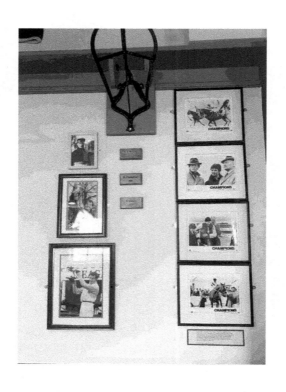

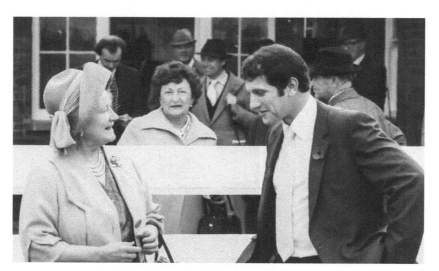

Against the Odds

I probably owe my life to a horse called Fury Boy and the fact he fell with me in a novice chase at Stratford on the evening of the 11th May 1979. If there's ever a story when what seemed like a bad thing turned into a good thing, then this is it.

It had come down to a two-horse race and I had the advantage by about thirty lengths. Fury Boy was running well and jumping easily over the fences, until the last. He clattered it, went down and I went out the side door. Only winded, I jumped up, looked back and saw that the distance between me and the only other horse still running, Truro, was so large I had time to remount. I made to grab at Fury Boy, but he kicked both hind legs out and caught me square in the nuts. Boy did that hurt! Don't ask me how I managed to stay on my feet or hang on to him, but I did. More staggering than running alongside him, I hauled myself up into the saddle, turned him to face the right direction, realised I hadn't got my feet properly in the stirrups but thought it would just have to do. We won by a full twenty lengths. He was my final winner of the season and brought my overall career wins up to 355. I wasn't to know I wouldn't be getting another one for quite some time.

In the immediate days following the kick one of my testicles had swollen, but rather than painful, it was just numb. I was like most blokes. I examined it with a bit of idle curiosity, wondered about it, ignored it mostly and after a night out with an old girl-friend, I was happy to know that everything was still 'working'. The season was over and I was going to head back out to the US like I had done the year before, but this time the trainers knew who I was and were already making enquiries about me. In fact, I was specifically asked over to ride Casamayor, the horse who I had pipped to third place in the Cheltenham Gold Cup, in an invitation race at the Hard Scuffle track. We finished fifth. After that, I went up to the stables in New York.

Yet again, like the previous year, I loved the variety the US offered. The quality of the training yards, the variation in the horses and the overall American lifestyle. It was so much more... I'm not sure of the right word. Not glitzy, but somehow more modern in comparison to Britain in 1979. Remember we had mass strikes, the TUC was in its ascendency, Scotland was voting for devolution, the IRA was conducting some of its most damaging attacks and Mrs Thatcher had just been elected for her first term. In comparison to the grey, washed out monotones of the UK, America seemed to be bigger, brighter, more optimistic. Their shopping malls were huge, their cars were superb looking, the gadgets in their houses fascinating, the weather was amazing and yes, the girls liked my English accent.

After a couple of weeks I joined up again with Burly Cocks in Pennsylvania and whilst it was a tough routine, it was a marvel-lous way of life. We worked hard and partied hard. 'Off-duty' ac-tivities included swimming, water-skiing, which I was okay at so I must have learnt something from Bob Davies during that time in Minorca, tennis and parties. A lot of parties.

Ironically, for what was about to happen, if you asked me to pick a month or two in my life when I felt vibrant, healthy, happy; more than that, content, then it was the June and July of 1979. I was loving the riding and, when I got a chance for a break, I had the USA spread out in front of me. Mexico too.

It was in Cancun, Mexico that I met an English nurse, Nicky Clapp. She was over there working on an exchange course from a London hospital. We'd meet up in the mornings for breakfast and at some point she mentioned that back in London she worked in a specialised cancer hospital. It was of passing interest at the time.

After that short break I joined Burly in Delaware. It was about that time that I began to get a bit concerned about my still sore testicle. I say sore, but it was just a bit firmer than the other and was getting gradually more numb. Fury Boy might have done a little more damage than I first thought and eventually, it must have played on my mind enough to overcome any embarrassment I was feeling, although I still couldn't bring myself to go to a doctor. Thankfully, a while before, I'd met a beautiful woman vet and we had started seeing each other. One night in bed I hesitantly asked her if she could take a look at it for me.

That's the thing I'd really like men to consider. I'd had this issue for ages but kept ignoring it, or more to the point, kept allowing my embarrassment to prevent me from seeking medical advice. For months I'd thought it would just go away. I mean, I could still 'perform' and to the male ego at that age, at any age, that's what was important. Yet even when my concern grew, I didn't ask for help. It's quite pathetic really and later on I would dwell on how much simpler my treatment would have been had I acted earlier. Saying that, had I acted even later there wouldn't have been any treatment, so I have to be grateful for finally speaking up.

It was the nagging doubt in my mind that forced me to seek another's opinion, but even then I almost clammed up due to awkward embarrassment, which is basically ridiculous. Putting it bluntly, I'd slept with this beautiful vet and you can't get more intimate than that, but I still found it immensely difficult to just ask her for some advice with regard to my nut. When I did, her reaction was stunning. In no uncertain terms she told me that I had to get back to the UK and get seen by a doctor. Immediately.

Over the years I've made a joke about that episode and how the key to good diagnosis is to date a vet, who after all trains longer than a doctor and is used to dealing with dumb animals who won't tell them what's wrong (like most men), but on the serious side, guys; GO GET CHECKED OUT. Doctors know exactly what to look for, after all, it's why they go to school.

If you think something isn't right, go to your GP. If you are at the age to have a regular prostate check, GO DO IT. Trust me, early diagnosis is going to save you a lot of discomfort and in fact, may well save you.

As for me, I flew back to the UK and was met by a long-time friend, Dottie Channing-Williams, who owned the Five Bells Pub near my house. It was in effect my local and I'd spent many a night in there, teasing Dottie that she should let me chat up her beautiful twin daughters. She never did. I had also come to trust Dottie and so I explained to her why I was back home. She told me to see a doctor as soon as possible. But still I dithered.

Although the delay allowed me to meet Sally at an event in the pub the following night. Poor Sally, who came into my life at a time that was about to get very complicated. She was a beautiful red-headed girl and had she known what was going to be coming our way in the next few months, she'd have run a mile. As a support to me she was wonderful, but I don't think she got or saw the best of me in return.

I did nothing about the doctor on the Sunday, but on the Monday I was to meet Derek, who was commentating at the International Horse Show in Wembley, London. I thought as I was in town, well what harm could it do, so I rang Dr Alun Thomas at his Park Street Surgery. Dr Thomas was the man I'd gone to see about the strange lumps under my nipples. As I've mentioned before, he was also the go-to doctor for all of us jump jockeys. He had patched, stitched, pinned and fixed more bits of riders than anyone else in the country. Given his standing in the medical community, he also had quite a few contacts and strings that he could pull. In the long run, that was to prove a major contributor in ultimately saving my life, for as soon as he got involved, the wheels weren't just put in motion, they were flying.

I stood in a proper red telephone box, rang him up and explained about the swelling, "Can you fit me in today?"

"Umm, I'll ring you back Bob, give me ten minutes."

I didn't think too much about it, loitered around the red box and sure enough, within ten minutes he rang back to inform me that he had arranged an appointment at a specialist hospital in Fulham

Road, Chelsea later that day. Now, had I made the appointment, I'd probably have cancelled, but because he had done that for me, I felt honour-bound to attend and duly made my way there by cab. I didn't even know the name of the place, just the address. Following a lengthy examination I was asked to come back an hour later to have another specialist take a look. The doc hadn't seemed that bothered, so I wasn't that fussed and wandered off to do some shopping.

On my return, still feeling fairly comfortable about the whole thing and curious about what they were going to tell me, my world was flipped upside down. The two doctors said they thought I had a tumour on my testicle and wanted me to come into the hospital the very next day. I'd be operated on, just as an exploratory, but there was a chance that they might have to remove one of my testicles for further tests. It could help in determining what type of tumour it was.

I was stunned. In my head I managed to translate what they'd said into, 'You want to cut off one of my nuts? Are you insane?' As it was, I said nothing. I think I was in shock.

They told me to go home, pack a bag and come back the next day. I walked off in a bit of a daze and that's when the full force of it all came crashing down on me. You see, to that point, no one had mentioned 'Cancer'. So it hadn't registered what I might be facing, other than the trauma of potentially having one of my nuts removed, but as I got to the main exit, I noticed the Hospital's name plaque; The Royal Marsden. It was where Nicky, the girl I had met in Cancun said she was based. It was a cancer specialist hospital. The realisation stopped me walking. It was a physical blow, like landing on the ground after a rough fall. I rationalised it, thought about it, twisted it and turned it as I meandered like a lost soul around London for a few hours. 'Don't be daft, Bob,' I thought. 'You don't have cancer. You're a fit and healthy jockey.' But the thought of having anyone operate on my nuts wasn't filling me full of confidence.

Derek and I had arranged to share a room in a hotel, so I ended up back there, but when I walked into the foyer I spotted the bar and headed straight for it. Now, as I've mentioned, I'm not a big drinker, but that afternoon I got stuck right into it as that seemed like the sensible thing to do. Honestly, I was a walking stereotype for most men. Deny the existence of the problem, and when finally faced with it, get drunk. Talking about it seemed to have passed me by. It began to wind its way into my head, over and over. What if, what if, why bother? I kept drinking, waiting for Derek to come back from Wembley. Then, as I downed yet another drink, I decided to go up to the room.

In my head I was going up for a shower, but when I got there it felt like the coldest, blackest, least hopeful place on the planet. I felt it inside of me. What was the point, if this was going to be cancer, then seriously, what was the point? No one survives cancer. Every ounce of my natural optimism deserted me. It was over. I was over.

I rang my sister, Mary to tell her I was going to jump out of the hotel window. She argued with me, told me to hang on, told me not to be so selfish, stupid, despairing. Basically she said anything to try to get me to snap out of it and I heard none of it. I hung up, walked to the window and discovered something about myself. I might have no fear riding at full gallop on a sixteen-hand horse. I might not even have any fear falling off that horse at almost thirty miles per hour, but it turns out I'm very scared of the thought of stepping out of a sixteenth-floor window. It's high. I remember thinking, 'That's a long way down and that's quite a bit of time to be realising you didn't want to do it.'

Thankfully, the moment passed, I had a shower, got changed and went back to the bar. Derek arrived and finally I talked. I talked to my best mate and explained my emotions, my fear, my worries, the feelings about being tortured with something I couldn't understand. We talked late into the night and I owe him a lot for that conversation. Later I went to the hotel nightclub but realised after only a few minutes that it wasn't a distraction I needed. I went back to the room, where Derek was already in one of the twin beds. I woke him up and started talking again. Telling him of the suicidal thoughts I'd had earlier. Then those very same thoughts returned. I paced back and forth, contemplating ending it all. Eventually Derek sat up and said, "Look, if you're going to do it, could you just kick on with it, mate? I'm tired and want to go to sleep."

That was enough to see me through. Thanks Derek!

The next day I returned to the Royal Marsden and was put through a mass of tests, from bloods to X-rays that seemed to be non-stop. I felt like a lab rat. They kept me overnight so as to better prep me for the surgery in the morning.

That night in July 1979 is a long, long time ago now and looking back on events in your life, there aren't really that many you can recall in utter clarity without notes or reminders, but I re-member that night. The chances of me sleeping were nil and all I could do was lie awake and think of the surgery the next day, would I waken with one ball, two, none? What would happen to my ca-reer, my future, and, if this was going to be cancer, what realisti-cally were my chances? Would I survive?

The following morning I discovered another thing about my-self that I hadn't known. When I became scared, really scared, I became belligerent. Those poor nurses were subjected to a whole argumentative tirade from me before, thankfully for them I imag-ine, the sedatives took effect and I was rendered unconscious.

As soon as I woke up in post-op recovery I raised the sheets and looked down. I had a scar on my stomach which was confusing. The doctor came in to see me and I was told that yes, they had removed one of my testicles and no, it wouldn't make any differ-ence to my 'performance'. However, the tissue samples were being sent off for testing and they would then know if it was benign or malignant. Either way, I wouldn't be riding for a good few weeks.

My good friend, Jonathan Powell, who would go on to co-write my first book with me, rang Josh to tell him I was in the hos-pital. I later spoke to Josh and told him I'd probably miss the start of the next season. He thought I was still in the US and responded with what would have been a really good joke, normally. "All those girls Bob? Have they finally decided to geld you? Haha."

I thought I'd better start at the beginning and when I had brought him up to date and that yes, in fact they had semi-gelded me, poor Josh was mortified. I even managed a smile at his apolo-gising over and over.

After the call I looked around and determined that I needed to get out of the Royal Marsden as soon as possible. I should say that jump jockeys, more than most, know the inside of hospitals. We have medical files that would make the average person double-take. The number of bones we've not broken is often less than those we have. For most, a season without at least one major break, fracture, heavy concussion or severe injury would be the exception. So you'd think we'd be comfortable in their surrounds, but I hated hospitals. I made it my mission to escape as soon as I could. I badgered the nurses and eventually, probably out of sheer frustration with me, they agreed to me discharging myself a full two days early, but only once I'd been to the outpatient department for yet more tests.

Thirteen days after the surgery I was called back to London. The tumour had been malignant and I owed a debt to Fury Boy and that kick of his, for highlighting what had already been there, invisibly killing me. However, not only had the tumour been malignant, but there was a shadow on the chest X-rays. The doctors wanted to take a closer look and it meant another exploratory operation. I became increasingly annoyed. I'd already missed the first week of the season and was ready to get back to racing, but I was told that they needed to do it as my test results had thrown up an anomaly. Normally a malignant tumour in the testicles would have spread through to the lymph nodes near the kidneys, enlarged the glands in the abdomen and then, eventually, spread to the chest. In my case I had none of those symptoms, except this shadow on the chest X-ray. I figured that further operations weren't necessary as the shadow was just likely to be left over from a previous injury.

I asked them what the surgery involved. Was it just an 'open me up and have a quick look' sort of thing? I was told that no, it wasn't. They would have to remove part of my rib to get to the centre of the lymph gland they needed to biopsy. That would be sent away for a comparison to the tumour on my removed testicle and then they'd know what we were dealing with. Funny enough, I'd had a few broken ribs and the pain is excruciating, so I wasn't looking forward to waking up after someone had removed part of one.

To be honest, I didn't want to be messing about with any of it anymore. Like a small child with a favoured activity, I just wanted to be back to racing. Eventually though I agreed to it, went home, packed another bag and returned.

On the 8th August I had the chest surgery and woke to see a variety of tubes coming out of me, including a chest drain. I was scared again and this time my belligerence was directed at the ones who meant the most to me, Mum and Mary. I know I took all of my fears out on them and I'm ashamed to say I really didn't behave well. Those who love us often bear the brunt of our anguish and this was one of those situations. Mary isn't one for taking nonsense but she knew me well enough to know that I was lashing out in fear. My Mum, always a gentle soul, was devastated that nothing she said could take the hurt and anguish away from her boy.

Of all the times I have looked back on those days, that lashing out at the ones who so dearly loved me, causes me the most regret. I was lucky that I got to apologise to them for my words and behaviours. But still… It's not a pleasant memory to reflect on.

During my recuperation, Josh came to see me. He was accompanied by a young owner called Henry Pelham, and a large bottle of brandy. While the nurses were off in other places, we demolished the bottle between the three of us and I discovered the mark of true friendship and loyalty. Josh knew that one of my biggest fears was that he'd replace me with another leading jockey.

He said, "I know racing's a cruel game, but I couldn't be like that. We've had some good seasons together, Bob. Your job will be waiting, however long it takes to get back on your feet." Now at that moment we both thought it would be weeks, maybe a month or two, and I really appreciated the sentiment. No one, neither Josh nor me, nor anyone else could have known how important that promise was to become. How pivotal it was to be in my life.

Despite Josh's commitment, I woke up the following day feeling miserable and it wasn't all to do with the brandy. I thought I'd go for a wander and that's exactly what I did. In fact I wandered right out of the hospital and found myself in a busy London street in my gown and slippers. The medical staff were not impressed when I eventually made it back. I got into another argument with a doctor who said that they had a duty of care to me and the least I could do was cooperate but, if I insisted on being childlike, I could just as well go home. So I did.

I was past caring at that stage and just wanted to start riding again. I know I was being awkward but they didn't see the jockey, they only saw a patient. Well, this patient had discharged himself early after what I considered were far worse injuries. In my head I had convinced myself that this was minor in comparison. I had totally convinced myself it was NOT going to be cancer. No way.

After a completely miserable weekend spent at home with poor Sally, she drove me back to the hospital. Again I was bad tempered and again she took it all without much of a word. I've never been a patient man but these were not good days and I'm pretty sure I would have driven Mother Theresa to frustration!

I sat in a small room waiting to hear what the results of the tests were. When I think back, I can describe that moment and that room in clear detail. I can see it in what we'd now call high-definition. But on that day, as the doctors began to speak, all I heard was that I had four or five months to live and I might not be able to ride again. Everything else faded away to grey and black.

Following the discussions, debates and arguments with Doctor Jane and her colleague, which I've already told you about at the beginning of this book, I finally gave in and agreed to start the treatment.

It was Monday the 13th August 1979. Day Zero.

φ

From me saying okay, I didn't realise how quickly everything would begin. First I was transferred to the Royal Marsden's Hospital at Sutton, Surrey and taken to their sperm bank facility to leave a sample. They'd already told me I could potentially be made sterile by the drugs and this was a way to preserve some sperm that might be used later, if and when I wanted to start a family. The thing is, the drugs I'd had prescribed and those first two operations had knocked me about so much already that the sample wasn't viable. I was caught in two minds. I might not make it through the treatment so what did it matter anyway, and another deeply sad-dening realisation that I might never have kids of my own.

From there they took me to a small room and started another series of tests. I was poked and prodded some more and then they sent me to a ward to wait. Thankfully, Sally had stayed with me and it's a good job she had, for the ward they sent me to was a mistake. Instead of the cancer ward, I ended up sitting in the corner of an acute medical facility with seriously ill old men, all of whom looked to be near death. Of course I didn't know it was a mistake me being here, so I panicked. I made to leave on a number of oc-casions and it was only Sally that stopped me from walking away from the whole thing. Eventually, even she couldn't prevent me from heading out the door, but a nurse finally realised the mix up and I was sent upstairs to the proper ward. To be honest, it wasn't that much more comforting. Old and young this time, all bald, all connected to drips attached to metal stanchions. Some bare-chested with their operation scars showing like strange marks of a combat that I was about to undergo.

I don't mind admitting that by now, I was terrified. It was a fear borne out of not wanting to die, but also simply a fear of the unknown. I really had no clue what to expect. Thankfully, just as it was getting to epic proportions and I was thinking of doing a runner again, a nurse called Jenny arrived. She would be a great source of comfort to me over the coming months and that began now, as she casually chatted to me about what was going to happen. More talks with the doctor followed, then I was wheeled off to have tests on my kidneys. Apparently the Platinum they were going to give me in the chemotherapy was acutely poisonous. Better to kill off the cancer cells, but toxic, so importantly they would also give me lots of other fluids to flush out my kidneys. Once the results were through I was sent back to the ward and put into a bed. I didn't even have a chance to go back home. This was it. This was where it was all to begin. I was confused and frightened, like a child facing a dark unknown.

Chemotherapy – Round 1.
Day 0

At 10pm the nurse came and fitted a cannula into my arm. It was a permanent, hollow fitting that allowed drips to be connected easily. As a first step it wasn't sore, just uncomfortable and awkward. She hooked up a saline drip of salt and water and hung it on my own metal stanchion. I still had hair, but this was my first step to looking the same as the others on the ward. That metal stand was to be a constant, annoying companion. Wherever I went, the stand on wheels went too. The nurse left, telling me to try and get some sleep. I didn't get much. Maybe it was due to the drip in my arm. In reality I was just so scared. I'm talking about a fear that consumes you, that is on a loop in your mind. How do you face something that you don't understand, an illness that you can't see, can't even feel inside of you? How do you convince yourself that you can survive when all around you is death and the smell of poison? It's the fear that paralyses you even when all you can think about doing is running.

Day 1

They woke me early with an offering of a hospital breakfast which I picked at. Had I known it was going to be the last thing I would be able to stomach for days, I'd have tried to eat more, but as it was I pushed it around the plate, then pushed the plate away. A nurse and a doctor came in to see me at 10am. They had a small drip bag, much smaller than the saline one and told me it was my first course of liquid platinum. The smell of it was unusual that morning. It was not just metallic, but *intensely* metallic. You could almost taste it at the back of your throat. Unpleasant in the extreme. In truth, it reeked. In time, I would come to hate it. When they brought lunch in, I already felt nauseous enough to refuse even the menu.

Later that afternoon, they gave me an intravenous injection of something called vinblastine and replaced the empty platinum bag with another saline drip. Dinner was a non-runner. By now even the thought of food was making me feel queasy. I did manage to sip down some Tizer and a little Coca Cola, but that was it. My fear, had gained a new friend; anger. Anger and fear is a noxious combination that can make you behave in a way that is not 'you' and this was certainly the case for me.

Day 2

I slept a little, but couldn't face breakfast other than half a cup of tea. Then the day started over again. Now you'd call it Groundhog Day, but that film was years away yet and anyway, there was one change. After the saline was swapped for the platinum and I got my injection of vinblastine, they added a third drug into the mix. Bleomycin was administered, again through the cannula. I began to feel sick.

Then I really began to feel sick and started to throw up. Here my two teammates started to get into their stride. My anger was being driven by the fact that only two days before, I'd felt fine. I had been a fit and healthy man, in my mind at least, and now the hospital was making me ill. Looking back even now, and even though I know it to be irrational, it made no sense to me that the illness was not affecting me, yet the treatment was. I was fearful of what was going on inside me and it was insidious, like a parasite eating away, destroying me. Mounting fear and anger left me being a hellishly bad tempered, surly man.

For God's sake, I'd been fit and happy. Now these doctors and nurses with their drugs and injections were turning me into some sort of human guinea pig. I convinced myself that it was all some sort of sick experiment. I know my mood swings were horrendous and yet again I have to think how mean, pig-headed and bloody-minded I must have been to those around me. But at the time, I couldn't have cared less. I was angry, I was sick and I was wondering if I'd survive this at all. In amongst this anger came a moment of light. Jenny came by and mentioned that a senior nursing Sister had specifically said she was coming in to see me later that day. I felt a little nervous, after all I hadn't been the best behaved patient so far. Well, you can imagine my delight to see Nicky, the nurse I'd met in Cancun just a few weeks earlier, walk through the door. She said she'd seen my name on the list and couldn't believe it was the same Bob that she knew. She reckoned

I'd looked so healthy back in Mexico. I felt a moment of peace for the first time as I knew that I would indeed be in very safe hands.

Day 3

The lady offering breakfast just walked away when I shook my head. Instead I was treated to another bag of platinum, but on its own. No accompanying injections. Feeling annoyed and angry and scared, I was certainly not amenable to company, but I remember that day I had the pleasure of some old girlfriends come visit. When you're this ill you don't really want company, I think I managed to be "sociable" for little more than fifteen minutes and that was when I was at my best.

On reflection, it's probably just as well I was grumpy. The first one left quite quickly, realising I wasn't my usual charming self and that meant she avoided the other one who turned up later. I did manage to break a smile that luck had helped avoid a bit of a potential embarrassment.

It was the only smile I was managing, for as well as the treatment, the nausea and the vomiting, I was becoming more and more worried about my finances. It's bad enough worrying about money when you are healthy, but I was getting seriously concerned at what was going to happen to me now that I had embarked on the chemotherapy. Some may have taken the blasé view of, 'why worry, I could die anyway', but that wasn't me. I wasn't going to die so I needed a way to pay my bills. My only source of income was gone, the Racecourse Compensation Fund wouldn't pay out because I didn't get the 'injury' in a race and I didn't have my own insurance, because we didn't back then. That left the State Sick Benefit, which at the time was a joke at less than fifteen quid a week. So you can imagine the huge boost that I got when Lord Oaksey and Brough Scott came to tell me that the Injured Jockeys Fund would look after it all for me and I wasn't to worry. I found out later that it had been Jonathan Powell who had made the initial call to the Fund. They'd arranged a loan to be paid to my accountant who was able to look after all my bills. I can't ever thank them enough for what they did for me. It was such a weight lifted, but sadly it didn't stop the ever-increasing vomiting that was taking hold of me.

Day 4

By now I was used to the familiar, but in between the drips and injections, the meals refused and the bouts of vomiting, the nurses would come and talk things over with me. It began to make such a huge difference to me. They explained what exactly a 'stage three testicular tumour' was. I understood the usual ages of men who got it; twenty to forty. I had the statistics explained; two percent of cancers were that type, but it was the second most common cancer in young men. I had the galling news that had I been diagnosed earlier, I could probably have had it beaten with a simple course of radiation therapy. But I was way past that.

The cancer ward's Sister, Carol, with Jenny from before, spent a lot of time encouraging me and the other patients to talk. In return I bombarded both women with questions. I wanted to know everything about the disease. How and why did a *teratoma*, the proper name for what I had, come to divide and double in size every twenty to twenty-seven days? Why was chemotherapy the best way to kill it off? How come cancer cells divided so much more rapidly than normal cells? How quickly would this work? How did it work? I pestered and pestered and was told by Carol, much later on, that it was a good thing. I was expressing my doubts and fears. I was talking through it. She said that the hardest patients to deal with and those who found it most difficult to cope, were the ones who bottled everything up tightly inside of themselves. No fear of me doing that. Questions and vomit. They both poured out of me. But those nurses were terrific. They understood the heavy weight of emotions that lay over us. They'd encourage us to ring them if we had any questions when we were back at home. I mean we had the doctors' numbers too, but I guess the nurses just saw more of what went on in the wards and had more experience, day in, day out of what those drugs could do to you. It's impossible to praise them enough.

Day 5 and Day 6

More platinum and vinblastine and bleomycin. No food, more vomiting and a series of warnings from the doctor. The in-ward phase of this round of treatment was over, but the side-effects would be kicking in. A main one being constipation. Now, that sounds like a 'not too bad side-effect' and that's what I thought when he said it. I understood what he was saying, but didn't concern myself too much. I really should have. In the coming weeks and months, I would come to understand what pain constipation can cause, for we're not just talking about not 'going' for a day. We're talking about not 'going' for seventeen days. The other thing the doctor warned me about was that my resistance to infection would be lowered. I was given a letter to show any other doctor should I become ill and I was specifically warned about the dangers of septicaemia, or what I knew as blood poisoning.

However, the great news was, the first hospital stay was over. Sally came and picked me up and to celebrate we stopped in at the Five Bells on the way home and for the first time in days I was able to eat. Then, in the very best of my stubborn refusal to accept the state I was in, I insisted we went home to mine because I wasn't going to be a burden on anyone else. I even had plans to go to a charity cricket match being organised by Jim Old the following day, but by the early hours of Sunday, I was ill; really ill.

Day 7 - 21

I couldn't sleep, I was sweating, I had stomach cramps, I was vomiting. I had a massive ache in my stomach and felt like I could burst. It was horrendously sore. I'm told Dottie Channing-Williams came to see me at Sally's request, but I can't remember her being there. Apparently I wouldn't let them call a doctor, but I kept asking them over and over to help me. I'm not sure what I wanted them to do, relieve me of my pain or of my life, because at that point I felt like I wanted to die. By five in the morning I couldn't take it anymore and rang Mary. By nine, I was in the spare room in her and her husband Richard's farmhouse near Wootton Bassett and it was just as well because I was going downhill fast. The pain from the constipation was incredible. The hospital had given me Milpar, an awful liquid that was meant to ease it, but it didn't, so I found some of the laxatives I'd used previously to help me shed the weight.

They used to work almost immediately, but not now. How completely stupid of me to have even tried them! If you've ever taken laxatives you know how uncomfortable they can make you, the cramps that they give. This was added to the already horrendous pain and I really didn't know what to do with myself.

I know Mary was scared for me and called her local doctor almost every day. She was worried that I might just die right there on the farm. But, pain or no pain, I held on. Richard took me back to the hospital on day nine for another injection of bleomycin and the nurses gave me an enema to help with the constipation. It didn't.

Back at the farmhouse it became almost a joke. Mary's kids, Emma, who was seven and her brother Nick, six, would make a great fuss over me and everyone would ask, first thing in the morning, "Have you been?"

It sounds funny, but it truly wasn't. I'd go to the toilet and sit there with a copy of the Sporting Life or the Racing Post and wait and wait and try and try. I'd literally be sweating and straining but there was nothing. By now, although I was eating again, the food had nowhere to go, so I'd just regurgitate it back up after about ten minutes. Practically for most of the day, if I wasn't sitting on it, I was kneeling over the toilet and the pain was indescribable. I could use every metaphor or simile in the thesaurus and nothing would get close to what it felt like. A combination of a deep, deep ache perforated with a series of stabbing pains that wracked the body and sapped all your strength. Back ache, leg pains, unable to breathe properly with a chest that felt like it was being sat on and a headache that would stop a bull-elephant. I'd try to stand and it would almost make me collapse. I'd stagger from bedroom to bathroom and back again, flopping, exhausted into a bed that was useless for sleep because I gasped at the waves of agony coursing through me. It was horrendous. And then, on day seventeen, release.

Nick and Emma delightedly ran through the house yelling to Mary and Richard that, "Uncle Bobbie's been, Uncle Bobbie's been!"

The thing about my cancer treatment was, that for every small up, there would be a real downer. Just after the constipation cleared, my hair began to fall out. I felt real misery and despair when I woke up, raised my head and saw large tufts of hair all over my pillow. God that was heart-breaking. Your hair is on your face and up your nose and in your mouth. There is a moment, just a moment when you realise that you are about to become a bald shadow of yourself. It sapped another little piece of resolve. It chipped away another bit of being 'normal'.

But then you had funny moments. Obviously most of the racing fraternity knew I was ill, but a rumour spread around Brighton racecourse that I'd died and the Sporting Life prepared my obituary. Thankfully one of their reporters rang a few people before they went to press. Mind you, that's happened a couple of times in my life. Just recently, Wikipedia had me dead for quite a few weeks and it turns out that it is harder to correct modern day Internet stories than the odd rumour in 1979. Back then, when Terry Biddlecombe learnt about my demise and rang Mary's to pass on his condolences, he was able to set his mind at ease, albeit with a bit of a shock, when I answered the phone.

He wasn't the only one though, so I decided to put in an appearance to set the record straight. I convinced Bob Davies to take me to Fontwell at the end of August. I was meant to go back to hospital for another injection of bleomycin, but I told them I couldn't make it until the next day. It was rather like playing hookey from school. It sounds like a stupid thing to do now, but back then I was getting really annoyed that everyone was thinking I was dead. I wanted to show them I wasn't. Although the effort in going nearly put an end to me. I mean, I could hardly walk from the bedroom to the bathroom and here I was going with Bob down to Josh's yard and then on to the races for the afternoon. It was madness, but it was also the day that I can point to and say, 'that was the day I really started to fight to survive.' I was damned if I was going to succumb to any disease and I was annoyed at people telling me I was dead. Mind you, some of my friends told me later that I had looked like death warmed up. They actually thought they were probably seeing me for the last time. For my part, I remember feeling cold, really cold and that was something that would be with me for the rest of the treatment.

Next day I had to go to the hospital for the last set of injections and surprisingly for the rest of that first round of chemo, I began to feel better. Still cold but able to get up and join Mary and the family in the kitchen. Mary, not one for letting me have it easy, would shout at me to get washed and dressed. It was her turn to be a bit of a bully to me, but she knew what she was doing, no malingering and it got me moving again. Of course my being downstairs meant I had access to the phone and the children nicknamed me, 'Tinkle Tinkle Bob' as I was always on it. Recalling this with Mary recently she reminded me that during my treatment I ran up a £1,000 phone bill! That would be about £4,000 nowadays. I must remember to pay her. *One day Sis.* Mary would also tell you that I had many a female visitor and so that they could keep up, the children would give them nicknames like, 'Smoke Salmon Jane' after one young lady who always brought me some! The children thought it highly amusing.

Mary's insistence for me to get up and about meant I started to eat and even managed to be well enough to borrow a car and drive to see Uncle Arthur and Auntie Eileen. I decided, that even though my hair was by now falling out in increasing amounts, I would attend the Christening of my friend, Jonathan Powell's daughter, Katie. I was to be her Godfather, which I think shows the faith that Jonathan had in me to survive when many didn't. I thought I was feeling better, I even thought the hair wasn't too bad. But again, in hindsight, I know a lot of people who saw me that day thought I looked gaunt, listless and terribly, terribly ill.

They and I, had seen nothing yet.

φ

Chemotherapy – Round 2.
On the 3rd September I started my second round of chemo and they'd already told me it would be worse than the first. Given how bad that first experience had been, I was petrified. If I'm totally honest, I didn't want to go through it again.

Back on a ward with others facing the same reality and waking that first morning to find even more lumps of hair on my pillow, I decided it was time to shave it all off. A nurse called Edna, who was quite the master with a cut-throat, shaved my head and face leaving only my eyebrows. God, it was depressing. It was like I had been marked out and boy did I fully realise just how vain I was. I didn't recognise the poor bald soul staring back at me from the mirror and in truth, I didn't want to recognise him. He wasn't me. He couldn't be. He was a cancer patient.

To help with the image issues, the NHS gave you a choice of wigs and you were allowed two. I took my first two and, over the weeks, managed to convince the supplier that a horse had eaten one of them. Not too sure he believed me, but I ended up with a total of four. One for day, one for the farm, one to sleep in and one for best. I used to hang them on the bedpost like some strange fur trapper's prize pelts.

I'd also make sure I had my wig on when anyone came to visit. Like I said, I was fairly vain, but it also allowed me to retain some form of inner dignity and peace. It's important to feel better even if only a little with regard to your appearance. It shouldn't be underestimated how big a thing a wig can be for a cancer patient. The only time I felt comfortable without a wig was on the ward, with the others. There was no room for vanity then. The real starkness of cancer couldn't care less about aesthetics. Also the ward was really warm and I was uncomfortable enough without adding a hot, itchy scalp.

I still had female visitors but these were becoming less and less. I wasn't in the mood for company and often the nurses would prevent women from seeing me. They thought the nurses were being 'job's worth' but it really was a kindness and the ward nurses never tolerated the 'Do you know who I am?' attitude from any of them!

Day 1 - 6

The second hospital session was truly awful. They'd been right. It was worse and because I knew what was coming next, it became atrocious. Hospital food was a complete non-starter and I could barely manage sips of water. I started vomiting early and sometimes would throw-up ten or twelve times... every hour. In fact I became quite the expert on what could trigger my sickness. From the sound of another patient being sick, to the horrendous smell of the platinum. Strangest of all the causes, was the very sight of one of the nurses. I'm not too sure what Freud would read into it, but there was one nurse in particular, really attractive and pleasant with it, but she only had to come into the ward and I'd be sick.

The doctors and nurses knew that I was having a much harder time of it with the vomiting than most of the others, but no one could ascertain why. It was just what it was and with such a new treatment there was still quite a lot of experimentation happening. Usually, being competitive by nature, if I'd been told I was more than the average anything, it would have cheered me up, but not in this case. In truth, I was still bloody annoyed at them for making me this ill, when before I had felt fine. So I continued to feel sorry for myself and stare listlessly at the hospital TV watching horse racing as and when I could. You'd think that would have cheered me up, but no, I had to make a downer out of that too, because Josh was doing really well in the new season and I knew that I could have been on a lot of those winners. As a result of all this, I became as miserable as a wet day on the Yorkshire moors. Add my temper into the mix and I really wasn't much fun to be around. The nurses must have been getting fed up, so they clubbed together to by me a 'happy hat!' I'd like to say I took it in good spirits and laughed and laughed and became the life and soul of the ward. But I didn't.

Because I was so low I needed something, anything, to help me rally at least a little. To help me feel like I was still in control of something. So I made myself go for walks. Everyone who goes through chemotherapy sets themselves a goal, a small thing that can be achieved. Well, that can be achieved on the good days at least. It's a way to judge your progress. For me it was sneaking out of the hospital and making it to the shop on the corner. They sold Ambrosia rice pudding in tins and I fancied this. I might have only managed a spoonful, but it served two purposes; it gave me something to get out of bed for and it meant I would eat just a little. The nurses would smile at me coming back with a tin in my hand.

Of course most of what I ate came back up. The anti-vomiting drugs didn't seem to work on me and neither did a drug called Largactil that was meant to make me drowsy. Because of that, my nights were mostly spent, between brief naps, looking up at the ceiling and focussing on the image of me and Aldaniti in the 1980 Grand National, only six months away. To be fair, at that point I didn't have the strength to sit on him for a minute, let alone ride him for four and a half miles over some of the biggest fences in horse racing, but the dream was worth hanging on to. Nowadays, you'd call it visioning or goal setting. For me back then, I never thought about it like that. It was simply my dream. My target. The thing that truly kept me taking whatever they were throwing at me.

I can also recall that my friends and family were so very caring and like most people when they visited a patient in hospital, they'd bring a gift. The thing is, without sounding mean, until you're in that situation you will never understand that the last thing a person going through chemo wants is chocolates or a box of cigars. But the thought was welcome and a lot of the hospital staff got some really nice gifts.

One of my visitors would be Josh, who took time out of what was a hectic schedule to come see me. His visits were always a source of strength for me and when he came I was always amazed at how upbeat, supportive and positive he was around me. Years later, when all of this was a bad memory, he confided in me that he used to dread going to see me when I was so ill looking and at no point did he expect me to pull through, let alone ride again. It hadn't helped him that a great friend of his had died a few years previously of cancer. He also told me later that quite a few of the owners had told him there was little chance I'd make it. Thankfully, Josh kept all of that to himself and only ever portrayed positivity when he sat next to my bed. I know now that he wasn't alone in dreading coming to see me and yet he and all those other friends and family still did. To be fair, I say I know now, but the truth is, I knew back then as well. They all thought I wouldn't make it and I could sense their fear and their sadness, but never once did a single visitor show me anything other than positivity.

For anyone with a cancer sufferer in their family or friends' circle, if you can, screw your courage to the mast and go see them. The boost they receive is amazing. Also, be forgiving. I was incredibly lucky, for no matter how cantankerous, belligerent or sombre I was, they still came and saw me through it. The power of their presence should never, can never, be underestimated.

Central to all of the visitors were my Mum and Mary; they were absolute rocks. Like Josh, always so full of hope and showing complete confidence that I would beat it. They were constants throughout my treatment as were Frank Pullen and Monty Court. They'd come most days when they could and cheer me up by talking about riding or just sitting with me. Frank was one of Josh's owners, but boy what an amazing life story that man had. Raised the youngest of four to a widowed mother in South London during the depression, he'd fought in the Second World War, survived the D-Day landings and came home to found a building company. A true example of the self-made millionaire who never forgot where he came from, he loved his horses and his cars.

Monty, the then racing editor of the Sunday Mirror, would bring me a copy of the Sporting Life and armfuls of grapes and bottles of various juices. I couldn't face most food and had barely eaten anything on this second round, but the fruit Monty brought helped take the sick taste from my mouth.

In the middle of all of this, I became slightly paranoid that the treatment I was being given wasn't actually needed. The fear I experienced at the beginning never went away, it simply shifted its form. It grew steadily and if I managed to defeat one bit then it would come back at me with something different. I now started to think they were using me as an experimental lab rat, or some strange science project for this new treatment regime. Because of that, I know I pestered the doctors and nurses so that I could see all my results. In fact, I demanded to know everything that was happening to me. I needed to see it in black and white, even the good news. When they said the tumour in my chest was shrinking I demanded to see the X-rays, because basically I didn't feel I was getting any better. My body felt like it was shutting down, not healing.

I recently went back over some of the paperwork that I'd been given at the time. It states; 'The expected side-effects of Platinum will include: Nausea, vomiting, anorexia, bone marrow depression, and numbness in extremities presenting as pins and needles.' Vinblastine was expected to cause the same pins and needles, anorexia, loss of weight and appetite and more bone marrow depression, which just means your blood cells stop producing, so no big deal. Finally, the Bleomycin only caused 'mild' bone marrow depression, but also came to the party with baldness, constipation, discolouration of skin, severe cramping and lastly, mouth ulcers.

I can, hand on heart, say that yes, I got all of those side-effects. Everyone and more besides. I often thought that I was actually in a race and it was even-money if the drugs killed off the tumour cells before they killed me. Of course, to combat all of that lot, there were side-effect controlling drugs, but like the constipation curing Milpar I've mentioned before, none of them seemed to work for me. Oh woe was me.

However, you couldn't get too self-pitying, for you aren't going through this on your own. There are other patients and one of them, diagnosed with the same type of cancer as me at the same time as me, was John Gobourn, a garage and plant hire owner from Wales. He'd originally been treated with radiotherapy, but it hadn't worked and after a second opinion found himself at the Royal Marsden. We became mates and would count the hours until we could get out. I think John coped with the treatment better than me, but he was a great friend and would help me get through the worst of it by talking about horse racing.

Day 7 - 21
Once the six days were up I was ready to go back to Mary's, but first I needed a hot bath. I've mentioned about the smell of the platinum on the first drip they gave me, but by now it would be seeping out of your skin and the stink was stomach churning. Like I said, I can't to this day describe it properly, it's just metallic but it's vile and in itself makes you feel sick. Think of the worst smell, the one you really can't stand and now imagine it, be it mouldy cheese, or a blocked drain or rotten fish, leeching out of your pores. Being the smell you reek of. It was horrible. You know, even now if I drive to Sutton I can smell it. I guess it's just in my head but it's as strong

as the days when I had my treatment and it never fails to make my stomach turn over.

To try to get rid of it, I'd always want a hot bath as soon as I was free of the cannula but I was usually too weak and would end up passing out. Luckily the nurses all understood the need for the bath and that they'd likely have to carry me back to the ward.

This time round there were to be no 'independent heroics'. I went to Mary's with no arguments and confined myself to bed for a week. By the second week I felt well enough to go downstairs and join in family life. The experience of the first time meant I knew not to eat too much. Even with control I still ended up in constipation agony, although it didn't last as long and I think after not eating for six days, save for a little rice pudding, it was a good sign that I could face food at all.

I spent a lot of my time at the farm reviewing old race tapes. Mary and Richard and even the kids soon got bored of watching me watching myself winning, but I found it a great comfort. It acted as a reminder of why I was fighting through all of this and it renewed my determination to race again. Plus seeing myself at my happiest and fittest helped to put aside the negative images and thoughts I had about myself. I believed that as I was half way through my treatment and that all the results were showing a marked reduction in the tumour, I could still be in with a chance of riding in the National the following spring. Josh had rung to say that Aldaniti was also back in training after his summer rest and would be looking to race at the end of November. There wasn't a chance in hell that I'd miss watching that race, I needed to see how he performed. Despite all the illness and the pain, the thought that grieved me most was that someone else might ride him in the 1980 Grand National. At some point around this time, the long suffering Sally said farewell. I couldn't really blame her. She'd put up with some considerable drama. Mary however was not one for my drama and if I so much as muttered, "It's ok for you, you're not suffering like poor me," she'd snap back with, "Oh yes poor, poor me."

I guess I didn't really expect sympathy and anyway, Mary knew sympathy was the last thing I needed. I needed to fight back against the disease. She wasn't about to see me feel sorry for my-self.

φ

Chemotherapy – Round 3.

On 24th September I started round three of the chemo and whilst I thought I knew very well what to expect, this time would be quite different.

Day 1 - 6

I went through the usual loss of appetite and vomiting, but the tins of Ambrosia rice pudding I brought in would be warmed in the canteen and it meant I could eat a little. It's funny that my memories of chemo mean I can no longer drink tea without retching at the thought, yet I still enjoy that rice pudding. Between the canteen staff, the porters and all the ancillary support staff, through to the nurses and the doctors, I was blessed to have been cared for by such an amazing team. No matter what you needed, the nurses would get it and if they couldn't, other staff would. There was a porter called Les, who liked a bet or two and therefore knew me. He'd go off and get me bottles of orange juice from the little shop and he'd pick up the pudding on the days I couldn't make it myself. Nothing seemed too much trouble and I know that back then and still now, hospital staff don't get the recognition they deserve. We laud pop-stars and actors and false heroes when these carers, nurses, doctors and porters truly are the real thing. Since those days I have been so lucky to work alongside the very best of the NHS and I am incredibly proud to be able to call so many friends.

Back then, on round three, I was still being buoyed up by getting regular visitors, including my Mum, Dottie Channing-Williams and of course, Derek. He would see me lying in bed feeling sorry for myself and bully me into getting up and exercising where I could. He'd tell me I couldn't let my muscles waste away, not if I wanted to ride again. I think he also wanted to keep me from spiralling too far down, so he'd make me get up and walk around the ward. It wasn't that big a space but it would take me almost five minutes with his help, then I'd collapse into bed again, exhausted.

He was such a positive support for me. I didn't know for years and years that he would go out into the car park and cry, thinking each time was probably the last time he'd see me alive.

During the weeks between treatments, when I felt a little better, he'd take me to the races for the day. It was hard going to be out and about, but again I was stubborn and determined to be part of my world. What I was less buoyed up by were the gifts that kept coming. Although they were no longer chocolates and cigars, now we had progressed on to books and food.

Both friends and public well-wishers, who were doing exactly that, wishing me well, would send me parcels. Their kindness is, from the distance of time passed, so much appreciated, but back then I couldn't face food and was too ill to read, so the constant gourmet offerings and boxsets of Dick Francis novels were not what I needed. Even when I was well I didn't read that much, so the books never got opened.

By now, past halfway through the expected four courses of treatment, my main concern was that the doctors still didn't know if I'd ride again. It wasn't their fault. I was the first professional sportsperson to go through this particular treatment so they had no way to know. Doctor Jane explained the potential drug damage to my lungs meant I could lose a third of their capacity. That was fine for the average person, but for me it could mean I wouldn't be able to ride to the highest standards. Again the fear whispered to me that I wouldn't ride, that I would never achieve my dreams. Frustrated, sick and tired of the whole thing again, on the 29th September I left the hospital with all the usual warnings. I just wanted to be out of the damned place, so I paid them the usual scant attention.

That was a mistake.

Day 7 - 21

Septicaemia occurs when a patients' resistance to infection and their blood count is at its lowest. In 1979 it would kill 2% of cancer patients. I very nearly became one more.

I'd been through the usual feelings of exhaustion, sickness and constipation only to wake on the 7th October feeling worse than normal. I didn't think that was even possible. I had mouth sores, then I developed spots and became more irritable than normal, if you can believe that and even snapped at my poor little niece, Emma. However there had been an escape of cows and Mary needed all hands on deck. I went out to help. In hindsight that was a mistake, and probably accelerated what was about to come. I was sweating and shivering and after a few pathetic hours trying to stay downstairs, I went back to bed at Mary's insistence. Later when she came to check on me she was concerned that I seemed to be burning up. She couldn't find a thermometer anywhere, so had to get a friend to bring one around. By that time I had a temperature of 102 degrees. Mary called her local doctor.

He arrived very quickly and after a brief examination called the hospital number listed on the paperwork I'd been given back at the start of my treatment. They advised that I should go to a hospital immediately. Although Swindon was closer, the staff at the Royal Marsden felt that getting me back to their care was vital as they were much better placed to treat me. Richard was still out in the fields and couldn't be found, so it was all getting a bit tense, although by now, I think I was well past caring.

When Richard did arrive and I was being carried out to the car, I asked Mary, "Am I going to die?"

"Don't be silly," she replied in her typical off-the-cuff way. "Only the good die young."

My sister. My Rock.

Years later I discovered that as I was being driven away, all of Mary's usual optimism and hope deserted her. She knew that she had quite possibly said goodbye to me for the last time. As we went out of sight, she broke down and was violently sick.

Now my brother-in-law is usually a sedate and careful driver but that night he became like Lewis Hamilton and it's a good thing he did. I was delirious and severely ill. He drove the 100miles to the hospital in a time that makes us grateful there were no speed cameras back then. The hospital were expecting us and there was a stretcher waiting for me as we pulled up.

The medics were as usual, brilliant. With a temperature now reaching 105, they gave me a massive dose of antibiotics and a blood transfusion. Within twenty-four hours my temperature was under control and I was out of danger. Later, the nurses told me I'd been about twenty minutes away from not pulling through. Strange then that my recollection of that evening was one of calmness. I had passed the point of fearing death. It was quite pleasant, there was no more pain and I can clearly recall thinking that it would be okay to go now. It would be peaceful and gentle to just slip away.

That night, the 7th October 1979, was a turning point. I'd never come as close to death again. Well, not for quite a few years anyway, but that's for later.

They let me home on the 12th for a short respite before what I thought would be my final course of chemotherapy. Monty drove me home in a car that barely went over 30mph and puffed out smoke the entire way. It was the tortoise to what had been Richard's hare.

At Mary's I can't remember a more emotional or warm welcome home. The septicaemia incident had scared us all more than we wanted to admit. From then on I did become a little paranoid and would insist on Mary taking my temperature far more than she needed to. I was a bit of a baby if I'm honest. If it was in any way raised, we'd check with the hospital. I'm glad to say the septicaemia never made a reappearance.

Chemotherapy – Round 4.

I had this licked. My last chemo session and then it would be me getting my fitness back again, me aiming to fulfil the goal of riding Aldaniti in next year's National. I wasn't thrilled at returning to hospital, but I wasn't dreading it either. One more go was all it needed, so on the 17th October it was 'ding-ding, round four'.

The biggest disappointment this time was it meant I would miss Derek's wedding to Jane McLaren. I was meant to have been Best Man and it was a huge let down not to be able to make it. Mind you, I think there was a small part of the happy couple that were vastly relieved, as my previous track record with weddings wasn't great. As the chief usher at a friend's wedding once, I'd given one half of the guests someone else's order of service and there was a proper old racket as the two sides of the church started to sing different hymns. So maybe Derek and Jane got off lightly.

I did send a telegram, which simply read, "I'm sorry I can't be with you, but I have to stay in hospital to look after the nurses." In his speech I know Derek said some very nice things about me and wished me a speedy recovery.

Day 1 - 6

Despite the fact I was in the last stretch, the six hospital days were as bad as ever. I was sick and weak and as the days marched by slowly I thought, 'That's it. When I get out of here, I'm never coming back.' Each of the preceding rounds had knocked me harder and harder and this one was a pummelling. All the side effects did their very best to hurt me. I couldn't eat, but I could still vomit. Well, I cramped terribly because I had nothing left to vomit, my skin oozed the metal smell of platinum, my body felt like it was being torn and pulled and pushed and crushed by some demonic giant child that thought I was a toy to torment.

And yet, in the midst of all of that, I managed to wind up my friend and fellow sufferer, John Gobourn. He just couldn't understand why, when we started our platinum drips at the same time, mine would always be finished first and I could get to leave almost a day ahead of him. On this fourth round I finally let him into my secret… The simple truth was I'd widened the valve in the drip so that the liquid would flow faster and the bag would empty into me more quickly. The nurses must have known, but I think by now they also knew just how much I wanted out of the confines of the hospital, so they turned a blind eye to it. Anyway, it cheered me up and meant they could get rid of grumpy Bob a day early, so it was a win for everybody.

I left hospital on the 22nd October having survived four courses of chemotherapy, the horrendous side effects and a bout of blood poisoning. I had also fought with my own demons of fear and anger and I'd won. My first re-assessment would be on the 29th November, but I reckoned I'd done it. I knew I wasn't quite out of the woods yet, but I thought I could plan for my recovery.

I was wrong.

Day 7 - 21

As usual, the first week was spent fighting off the side effects, so there was no chance of any celebrations, but by the start of November I was making massive improvements. By the 7th November I was well enough to drive and by the end of the 21-day cycle, with the last visits to hospital and the last injections completed, I was already feeling stronger.

Mary, Richard and the kids decided that they could go ahead with their long planned holiday to the States. I told them, and I really felt it was true, that I would be fine. I wouldn't be all on my own as I had a new girlfriend, so they should go, have a great time and not worry.

The day before they were due to leave, the 15th November, was a big milestone. I decided to get back in a saddle for the first time since July. Not a racehorse obviously, but my niece Emma's little pony, Henry. I'd been warned by the doctors not to bang my head as it would potentially be very dangerous, but they'd also encouraged me to get back to usual activities. To me, that meant riding a horse, so up I climbed onto the back of the 13½-hand pony. I walked him off, then tried a trot, then cantered round the adjoining field and popped over a couple of little tree trunks. I was delighted. Really chuffed. Mary thought I was mad, but she, Richard and the kids were all beaming up at me and then, as I got off, I nearly collapsed. I was completely knackered. My legs were wobbly and I was puffing like an old man. But... I'd ridden a horse again. It was just the thing I needed to do to prove to myself I was on the mend.

I drove Mary and the family to the airport next day and then went on to Ascot to watch Kybo, who I'd won the '78 Christmas Hurdle with and who'd now been swapped to fences, win a novice chase. He really was an amazing horse and Josh thought it might be the best he ever trained. Afterwards Richard Pitman, now retired and working for the BBC, interviewed me on air. I was far from looking ruddy and healthy, but I purposefully said that I was determined to be back in time for next year's National.

With Mary and the family away I began to get up and go for walks in an effort to begin the path back to full fitness. A week or so later I started riding out for Paul Cole down in Lambourn, but that was a bit too ambitious so early on. I wasn't fit enough yet and one morning after two other jockeys fell heavily next to me, with one of them badly hurt, I thought I better back it off a little.

On the 19th I had my first night out in a long time, attending the Stable Lads' Boxing tournament in London. This annual function always raised a large amount for the Stable Lads' Welfare Trust and I was really pleased to be there. Of course my metabolism was shot, so one or two drinks would have been an overindulgence and I may have had more than one or two! The following day I was due at the hospital for some blood tests, but I had to come back a day later, as my blood count contained too much alcohol to take an accurate reading. Oops.

All in all, I was feeling stronger as each week passed, but the worry was growing in my head. It was fast approaching time for me to go back to hospital for a full re-assessment.

φ

I stayed with the newlyweds, Derek and Jane the night before the re-assessment and in the morning, Derek drove me to the hospital. There, Doctor Jane started off by telling me how pleased she was with all that had happened. The tumour in my chest had gone. The treatment had been remarkably successful. I was to be congratulated for having come through it so well. Just as I was feeling on top of the world, she added… But.

"The thing is Bob, there are a few malignant cells in some fibrous tissue surrounding where the tumour was. We can kill those off with a straightforward course of radiation, however, the radiation and the drugs that accompany it, will absolutely diminish your lung capacity further than we already have."

"By how much?"

"It would be well beyond what you would need to go race riding again. I know you don't want that."

"I take it there's another option?"

"Yes. You'll need to undergo another two rounds of chemotherapy."

My world dropped. I had a shuddering pain sweep through me and it took all my concentration not to weep. It's hard for me, even after all these years, to sum up how I felt. I was truly heart-broken. I'd been so hopeful and buoyant as I walked through the door, believing that I had been getting my life back and now? I know, I know... If I wanted to give up the prospect of returning to the saddle I could have opted for the radiation, but I'd be buggered if I was going to drop my dream now. It was what had kept me going. Me and Aldaniti in the National. Yet I knew, with another two rounds of chemo, the chance of me riding at Aintree the following spring was becoming more and more unlikely.

My sorrow turned quite quickly to anger. Fine! Damn it and all of them! I'd take their bloody chemo again, and again. I went home and began to drink. Seriously drink, whatever I could get my hands on. I woke the next morning to one hell of a hangover and just about got myself together enough to go to Sandown. I met up with Josh and Nick Embiricos in the saddling enclosure. Aldaniti was returning to the track for the first time in the season, with Richard Rowe in the saddle for the Ewell Handicap Chase. At 3miles, 118yards it was an honest reintroduction to the track, not being too far nor too tough a test, yet I looked on dumbfounded as Aldaniti was pulled up, just shy of the finishing line, completely lame in the same leg as before.

The tendon injury he had suffered prompted the vet and Josh to both recommend that the old fella be put down. Thankfully, Nick and Valda recalled my long ago statement after the Silver Fox Chase, 'That horse will win the National one day,' and so they decided to get him treated and once again, confine him to box rest. They said they'd get him fit.

None of that mattered to me. I was numb. I couldn't believe what life was throwing at me. Even if Aldaniti did recover, there was no way on earth he'd be fit for the following year's Grand National. Not one chance. It was as if fate had decided to hand us both a crushing blow at the same time.

I was falling apart inside, but somehow, from somewhere, I drew on a reservoir of strength, or perhaps it was my bloody-mindedness in the face of increasing adversity. This was just one more thing to be overcome. I looked straight at Valda and Nick and said, "Never mind, we'll just have to come back together."

The truth was, I didn't believe it myself.

φ

I spent the next few days drowning my sorrows. I was lost. Completely rudderless and adrift in a sea of hopelessness. That may sound overly dramatic, but hope is all you have and mine had gone. All I had left was another eight weeks of misery facing me. Mary and the kids came home. It had just been Emma's eighth birthday, but my mood was infectious and no one seemed to want to celebrate. On Monday, the 3rd December, I went back to the Royal Marsden for the next round of chemotherapy.

Chemotherapy – Round 5.
I can't tell you why, perhaps it was my sunken mood, my disconsolate frame of mind, my feeling that this was all getting 'a bit too unfair'. Perhaps it was because my body had taken so much to this point. Whatever the reason, this session was by far and away the worst. I look back now and I can see that my bizarre dream of riding a particular horse in a particular race may have seemed a bit strange, but that vision, goal or target, call it what you will, had sustained me through the darkest of days. This time, that vision had slipped into shadow. I gave up my fight for a couple of weeks. The coming Grand National was an impossible dream. I wouldn't be riding again that season. I might not be riding ever again.

Day 1 - 6
All of that darkness contributed to me feeling as ill as I have ever felt. My veins were so badly damaged by the poison that trying to get a cannula in was a task that only the best nurses could achieve. We all used to dread the cannula coming out in the night because if a doctor had to do it you were in for a long and painful time. I vomited so much and retched so hard that I was racked with pains in my chest. I was forced to take sips of tea just to give myself something to bring up as the dry heaving was excruciating. The physical exertion of it made me sweat profusely and the platinum's

metallic stench poured out, causing me to heave more and more and more. To this day, because of that mix of smells and triggers, I can't drink tea without wanting to vomit.

My visitors kept coming, but I couldn't muster the strength or inclination to be in anyway positive. Even the normally funny and kind Frank and Monty couldn't raise me up.

Those two men were quite something though. They rang Josh and told him that they didn't think I'd last the week. I was feeling so sorry for myself that I pleaded with Frank to tell the nurses to let me die. He was really angry at me. He gave me such a mouthful about not having come this far to let all my friends and family down. I know he said it for effect, but I didn't even rally much at that point.

It's a strange time, when you are that ill. You really do find out about your friends and their determination to help you. Frank would sit with me, wiping my face when I was sick and emptying the bowl out, then returning to sit quietly. Just being there for me and with me. You can't ever repay that level of friendship.

Monty was the comic of the two. He'd always try to make me laugh, or he'd tell me all about the racing, but this time around, again with a finality and an undeserved bitterness, I simply told him to just go away and leave me alone. He didn't. He never took offence either. He just kept coming to see me, kept making jokes. Kept telling me about the races. He never told me what he was really thinking at the time; that I'd be lucky to survive and that he thought I'd never ride again.

Even the nurses were convinced that the lung capacity damage, just with the chemo and not the radiation, would probably stop me from regaining my career. All in all, it was a dire time. I started asking them to give me a break from the constant drips. I pleaded for them to make the gaps bigger and bigger. I couldn't take it anymore. I didn't want to take it anymore.

By the Thursday, I was finished. I couldn't go on. I summoned the ward sister, Carol and told her that I wanted off the drip permanently. It was over. I had reached the end of my tether and genuinely I'd had enough. I told her that I just wanted to go home to die and I meant it. Not in a dramatic or pouting way. I meant it as much as anything I have ever meant in my life. I was done.

Carol was an experienced ward sister. She'd seen it all before and wasn't surprised. She didn't even try to argue with me. All she did was suggest I take the drip off and go for a walk, have a think about it. She suggested we keep the cannula in, but when I returned, if I still wanted to stop, then she would agree. It would be over.

Free of the damned drip I wandered off and felt my spirits rise. I was released. I didn't have to suffer anymore. I could go out on my terms. I didn't care about letting people down. They didn't know how hard it was, how terribly sick I felt, how crushing it was to my spirit. No one knew. They couldn't understand and even if they did, they'd be unlikely to have coped with as much as I had. I'd done my best. Now, I was done with the lot of them. I could give in and be rid of the pain, once and for all. Within the midst of my despair, in a strange way, that thought of being finished made me happier. The cancer could do what the hell it liked. I was beaten. I'd happily slip away and stuff the lot of it. I look back and I know one thing for certain, had Carol argued to leave the drip in my arm that would have been it. I would, without a doubt, have gone home and I would have died.

To this day I have no clue how or why I took the path through the hospital that I did. Perhaps it was a guiding spirit, perhaps fate, perhaps pure luck, but whatever the reason, eventually, I found myself in the children's cancer ward.

Upstairs, in the adult ward, because we were all equally sick and miserable, we didn't tend to talk much. Even when visitors came in, if they weren't for you, and even most times if they were, we didn't really make an effort. But here, I walked through the threshold of the ward and was greeted with a chorus of 'Hellos!' and a flash of smiles.

I was bald like them, and was in a gown, like them, but I was bigger and a stranger and they thought that made me interesting. They came around and talked to me. Some of these little children were only three or four years old, all undergoing chemotherapy treatment. Most had cancer, in all shapes and forms, some had leukaemia. All were resoundingly cheerful! I was swept along by their resilience, their disposition, their… happiness. Yes, these little kids were bright and happy. What was happening was just happening. No big deal. They were coping. One little girl, about six or seven, her hair still not fallen out, but obviously receiving the early stages of chemo evidenced by the discolouration of the skin around her slightly sunken eyes, was gently moving back and forth on a rocking horse. She gave me quite a serious look and asked me why I was here.

"I'm just going for a walk."

"It's a nice hospital, much prettier than my last one," she said.

I think I smiled and agreed with her, as you do. Then she half tilted her head in the inquisitive nature of children and said without any embarrassment, "Are you going to die, or are you going to live?"

I know what went through my mind at that point, the myriad of emotions, the complex feelings that made me humbled to be in the company of these kids and, at the same time, ashamed of how I had said I was going to give up. It seemed to last for an age, but was probably only a second or two. I definitely know, that in the movie 'Champions' when they recreated this moment so accurately, John Hurt's acting genius was revealed to me in no uncertain terms. He managed, in just the look in his eyes, to capture everything I had thought and felt in that rarest of moments. Rare, because it was destiny changing.

"I'm going to live," I answered and in return I got the broadest of beaming smiles.

What a humbling experience. What a truly life-changing experience and one that I have never forgotten. I learned a very important lesson and an awful lot about myself that day, surrounded by those kids who were undefeated. There I was moaning at everyone, thinking only of myself, yet downstairs were those poor children going through the same without complaint! Seeing them was an absolute turning point for me. Leaving their ward with tears in my eyes, I resolved that if they could do it, then so could I. I knew that I had to return to Carol and I am a little ashamed to admit that I took the long route back, trying to think of what to say to her that would salvage at least a little of my pride. I need not have worried when, as I rather sheepishly asked her to put the drip back in, she just gave me a warm smile and said, "Of course Bob." For the rest of that stint, I took whatever they threw at me.

I was released from hospital on the 8th December.

Day 7 - 21

The routine was by now standard. For the first week, feel exhausted and sleep a lot. Eat food, get constipated. Revisit the hospital for the top-up injections, keep pressing through and as the 21-day cycle wound down, begin to feel marginally better. I began to realise, but cautiously after the disappointment of last time, that I was nearly there. They'd done their best to finish me off but under it all was a fighter and I wouldn't be beaten. Helped by some brave little battlers in a children's ward.

The only difference was that on the first Wednesday back home I was readmitted into hospital with a cold. Out of all of my stays, this one was quite fun. I didn't have a drip and I could meander about the place chatting as I went. After they were sure I was fine and that there was no danger of the septicaemia returning, I was discharged again. I arrived home to learn of an accident.

Four horses had escaped from a field on the farm and galloped into the main road. Poor little Henry, Emma's pony, had been hit by a car and killed. The other horses were fine, but as you can imagine Emma was distraught. For the first time in such a long time, I was able to provide some comfort and compassion to my niece, as she had done for me over those many months.

The sixth round of chemo was looming, but I asked the hospital if I could postpone it until after Christmas. They agreed. I'd start it on Boxing Day. They were flexible, but not slack.

That Christmas was a lot of fun, but it wasn't all smiles. On Christmas morning I'd woken up with swollen breasts. I was terrified. Mary of course decided that this was a great way to tease me and pointed out that I'd obviously started turning into a woman! As it was Christmas we decided not to go back to hospital until my scheduled date and so it was a worrying couple of days but ones full of love.

My parents had come to stay and it was wonderful to have all the family around. For a grown man, I didn't half get a lot of presents that year. I think anyone that knew me sent me something as a token of affection and a nod to the fact I was still here. However, what Josh Gifford sent me was far from a token. I opened an envelope to discover he had gifted me £1,000. That was a lot of money back then and so typical of the man's generosity. He'd promised to keep me on and he'd promised to pay me my usual retainer back at the start of the illness, but he'd also written to all of his owners and collected up about seven hundred quid. Then he topped it up himself. That was Josh all over. God, I look back and think how amazingly fortunate I was to know the people I did.

I also got a card from Aldaniti! Well, I got a card sent by Alexandra Embiricos, the young daughter of Nick and Valda. She'd created an Aldaniti fan club with several of her friends and charged a small subscription. The money they'd raised was included with the card and there was a note asking if I could donate it to the Injured Jockeys Fund. It was a sign of that girl's nature as Alex, who became an accomplished jockey winning fifty-plus races in point-to-point and under rules, still raises money for good causes and to this day sends a donation to the Injured Jockeys Fund each and every Christmas. In 2010 she cycled from Land's End to John O'Groats, raising over £10,000 pounds for the Bob Champion Cancer Trust. Overall she's raised many thousands of pounds for it and recently became a Trustee of the Fund.

With those type of people in your life, it's hard not to be upbeat, so I returned to hospital on the 26th December, in good spirits and ready to face my last treatment, even though I was still worried about the swelling in my breasts.

Chemotherapy – Round 6.
Day 1 - 6
The swelling turned out to be a reaction to the injections and nothing untoward. If I had contacted the hospital over the Christmas period I could have had my mind put to rest. That good news was a good start and I don't know if it was my mood or if finally I was

catching a break, but this stint of in-ward treatment was the absolute easiest. Although I think I really have to credit it to the dedication of the ward nurse, Jenny.

She had been getting increasingly annoyed and frustrated that every counter-side-effect drug I had tried, had failed. She was determined to find something that worked. Immediately on my return back on to the ward, she tried another drug that was given to the kids.

"You'll be out like a light, Bob."

Sadly, I wasn't.

Not to be put off, she mixed another concoction.

"This time, Bob."

She'd barely finished the sentence and I was asleep. At last! A drug that would knock me out while I was having the chemo administered. I slept so well that I was hardly awake to be sick. Even when awake, I was drowsy. It made the days on the ward fly by.

It seemed everything was on the up and up until, on the last day, the swelling under my nipples came back. I felt my stomach lurch and almost broke down. The doctors immediately rustled up a set of tests and I waited in a mild state of panic to discover if the cancer had spread again. Thankfully, the bloods revealed it was just a side effect of the drugs. Strangely they remained swollen until the summer, then they returned to normal.

And then it was over.

I left the Royal Marsden Hospital at the end of my last in-hospital treatment on New Year's Day 1980. It seemed lucky to me. New year, new start.

Day 7 - 21

If this stint had been the easiest when on the ward, it was by far and away the absolute worst when I was released back to Mary and Richard's farm. I was ill, constipated and more than any of that, I was weak to my core. I couldn't walk from the bedroom to the bathroom without being exhausted. My muscle definition had completely gone and when I looked in a mirror an old, wasted, shadow of a man looked back at me. I was meant to return to the hospital on day nine for my usual follow-up injections but I was literally too weak to travel. Two days later I was just about able to return and have the injection of bleomycin, but the staff decided I wasn't strong enough to have the rest of the blood tests done, so back home I went.

It's a strange feeling, knowing that you are the same person inside your head, but your body is letting you down. Weakness is a horrible feeling when your mind is as strong as ever. I hated it. To put what I'm saying into context, you have to understand that I wasn't just tired or lethargic, I was so weak that I couldn't go to the toilet on my own, or wash myself. I was like a baby having to be tended to and cleaned a few times a day. Adding to the physical deterioration was my anxiety and downright fear of what would happen at the first re-assessment. I doubted I could go through anymore chemo. It had taken all that was left of me. Now just to be clear, this wasn't a will power issue. The kids on their ward had 'cured' me of feeling sorry for myself, no this was a purely physical thing. I couldn't see my body surviving another session or two.

A couple of days passed and I went back to the hospital for the blood tests. It perked me up quite a bit to know that, so far, all was good. The staff kept telling me to give it time.

A couple of weeks more and sure enough, I was able to walk around the farmhouse. Well, for a few minutes anyway, then I'd be sleeping again. Mary and Richard both insisted that I not overdo things and I'd listen to them, but I found it increasingly hard to listen to friends that were telling me I should really think about a new career. Jump jockey was no job for someone who'd survived cancer apparently. I just ignored anyone that was telling me that. Politely, but ignored nonetheless. I was going to ride again. I even contacted the Jockey Club early on to advise them I'd be wanting my licence back. I suppose they could have ignored me in turn, but they didn't. Peter Smith, who was a long time mainstay of the organisation, immediately said that they'd back me and return my licence as soon as I felt fit enough to do it justice.

It seems a small thing, but it was small victories like that which allowed me to keep going. Small incentives and targets were becoming important. As soon as I felt a bit stronger, I decided to jog to some cottages that were about 100yards from the main farm-house. Well, I say jog, it was closer to a shuffle in my slippers, pyjamas and dressing gown, but it was more than a walk around the living room and so that made it a new, bigger, braver goal to achieve. It was where I had to start.

In the third week of January 1980, I went back to the Royal Marsden for the last set of injections. After this outpatient visit, my only other visits would be for the re-assessment and then the array of tests and checks they would put me through every month for the foreseeable future. As Richard was driving me back to Mary's I made a promise to myself. No matter what the outcome of the next re-assessment was, I had done my lot with chemo. If I wasn't cured by now with the drugs they had given me, then it wasn't meant to be. I'd never have chemotherapy again.

I never did.

A Stayer's Hurdle

My re-assessment would be on the 31st January. Until then all I could do was begin the long road back to fitness and of course… worry myself into a state. The former was positive, the latter inevitable.

I contacted Val Ridgeway, the remedial masseuse at the Hungerford Squash Club. She had helped me in previous years after heavy falls, but when I went to see her this time she couldn't hide the look on her face. I suppose I'd gotten used to my appearance. She hadn't seen me since I was ill and didn't manage to mask her shock at my wasted muscles and emaciated state.

Thankfully, she decided that this sack of skin and bones could be helped and set to work straight away. The deal was that I would exercise and she would massage and manipulate me back into a reasonable state.

On the 24th I was called back to the hospital for interim blood tests, a full body scan and the vital lung function tests. The doctors had told me that the bleomycin could have seriously compromised me and whereas most patients would be content with their cancer having been eradicated, I needed to make sure I had enough breath to be able to ride again. I was exhausted by the time the tests finished, but once more, it was a case of so far so good.

Returning to the farm, I decided that I would move back home. I knew I had to stand on my own two feet again and the sooner I struck out independently, the better. Staying with Mary and Richard would have been the easy way out and I couldn't do that. I also hadn't been in my house for months, so I was keen to see it hadn't gone to rack and ruin.

I do need to make this quite plain though; reminiscing about those months has brought to the fore all of the emotions I felt at the time. I knew then, as I still know now, there is no way, not a single hope, that I would have made it through my chemo treatment without the love and support of Mary, Richard and the kids. I can only hope they know how much they mean to me. It's especially important for me to thank Richard properly. Mary was my sister and the kids just had to go with the flow, but Richard had all of their emotions to cope with as well as helping me with my illness. He was such a strong force and held it all together, as well as turning into a racing driver when required. He was brilliant. So I wasn't moving out because of them, I was returning home because I felt it would be another 'kick up the backside' to get me back on my feet.

I also wanted it done five days before the re-assessment so I could start concentrating on my fitness from then on. What would have helped with my new regime was a full night's sleep, but as the 31st got closer and closer, I was sleeping less and less. Those last nights were spent lying awake and worrying.

The big day came and I drove myself to the Royal Marsden. I needed to do this on my own. It's no surprise and I can freely admit, I was terrified at the prospect of them telling me I needed more chemo. I was sure my mind was strong enough to take it, the kids in the ward had made sure of that, but I doubted my body could have withstood another round. As it was, I needn't have worried.

Doctor Jane looked at me and said, very simply and with no outward show of emotion, "The cancer's gone, Bob."

The feelings that rushed through me were hard to explain then and it's still difficult now. Relief certainly, and a profound sense of gratitude for all the staff that had treated me and helped me. A wave of love for my family and friends that had seen me through it and… and something else. A strange mix of being humble that I had made it and a shuddering, earth-shaking conviction that I needed to prove to everyone I was worthy of this second chance. I had to show the medics that their skill and devotion meant something. I had to show my family and friends that their love had mattered. I had to hope that the powerful guilt I felt at having survived when so many others hadn't, including some of the children who had given me so much resolve, would lessen over time. I figured that if I could fulfil the promise I'd made to myself, then I'd be able to prove to everyone their support had been worthwhile. I'd damn well be a professional jockey again. Nothing was going to stop me.

I ran to my car, drove to the nearest phone box and rang my Mum, then Mary and a few close friends. I think they could tell how fantastic I felt. Yes, I'd need check-ups for the next few years, each and every month at the beginning, but I couldn't dwell on a relapse. I was cancer-free and that was that. On the drive back home I think the full weight of how lucky I'd been hit me. You may say, 'Lucky, what on earth was lucky about getting cancer?' But I had been lucky. It had been caught, just in time maybe, but caught. Had I contracted it five years, maybe even two years earlier, then there would have been no recovery. I'd have died, simple as that, but the research and advances in that time had made a huge difference. Not that I realised it then, but perhaps a small seed was planted.

My next goal was to get fit, but first my good mate Ian Watkinson and I were going to go on holiday together. Ian was noted in racing for seemingly being impervious to pain and for having ridden some of the great horses of the time in the shape of Tingle Creek, Night Nurse and the phenomenal Sea Pigeon. Sadly, his career had ended at the final ditch at Towcester when he took one fall too many and suffered severe head injuries. Both of us had agreed that as soon as we were adequately recovered from our ailments, we'd be off to the sun.

Well, by mid-February we both thought we were good enough and off we set for Miami. No plans other than the flights and a hope to hit the road in the 'Sunshine State' and have some fun! What a disaster. The flight time was much too long for me and I was suffering when we landed. We had to find the nearest airport hotel just so I could recuperate. The next day we headed for Miami Beach and all the wonders it would hold. It turns out that in Miami at that time of year there is no one under the age of about seventy-five and every single hotel room that you would want to stay in was fully booked. We ended up in a flea-pit and would go for walks along a geriatric beach before heading back to the room to watch mindless TV. Still bald, I'd leave the wig off to see if I could get a bit of colour into me, but was then asked if I was a member of a religious order. All in all, it was awful. We pulled the plug after four days and headed home. Obviously, I blame Ian and as I see him regularly I can and still do wind him up about it.

Although there was one high spot. In the taxi on the way back to the airport, we goaded the driver to go faster and faster. Teasing him about being slow and cautious he kept putting his foot down more and more. Eventually a cop car came pursued us, pulled us over and issued our unfortunate driver a ticket. By way of amusement it was the only thing that cheered Ian and me up. Those American cops do have pretty big guns and it was just like the TV shows.

Back in England I realised that to get fit I'd need more than Val helping me. If I wanted to be properly 'Jockey Fit' I needed to be riding horses. It's like a football player only being able to get 'Match Fit' with game time. But to be able to ride at all, I needed a latent level of fitness first, so I enlisted the help of a guy called Pete Fisher, another member of the Squash Club. He was an all-round athlete and a very good football player. The first thing he got me doing was running and the first decent run, of just two miles, nearly destroyed me. But the next time was easier, as was the next and it came down to how much did I want to improve. The answer was, a lot.

As the end of February approached, my sleepless nights started again as the next set of tests loomed. Once again, my worry was for no reason. All was well, in fact better than well. The doctors said everything was perfect. I breathed a sigh for another four weeks. Within which time I started riding out again. Not for Josh, but for Paul Cole. At first I walked the horses, then trotted, then risked a canter or two. Paul was very accommodating and we both knew that I was far from being able to ride a full-blown thoroughbred properly, but he kept letting me ride out and I kept turning up every morning. Then I'd report to Val who would help me recover, then I'd run. Sometimes I would go back to Val again on the same day. On as many days as I could, I would go to the race track.

Between all of these activities I was discovering some interesting things. My hands were almost constantly numb and I had little feeling in my feet. That made the whole task of holding reins and controlling a horse a bit of a tough job. Although mostly numb, strangely my feet ached and the more tired I would get the dizzier I would feel. Like I was off-kilter, out of balance. Worst of all was my back. It would ache during the day and go into spasms at night. The only thing that kept me focussed was the sure and certain knowledge that if I stopped, it would get worse. I had to get fitter, so I had to keep riding and running and being as active as possible. I suppose some may say I was quite determined and I know there were things written in the past about that, but for me it wasn't a commitment or a determination. It was just what I had to do if I was to get back racing. So I just got on and did it.

Of course I'd also been to see Josh and we both agreed that the earliest 'comeback' I could realistically aim for would be the start of the next jump season, at the end of July.

You may be reading this and thinking, 'that's good', but I'm not sure I have managed to adequately express the incredible thing Josh Gifford had done for me. He was a trainer and trainers are not responsible to jockeys. They're responsible to the people who ultimately pay their wages, the owners. Owners invest a lot, and I mean A LOT, of money into horse racing, so they expect the trainers to be doing their absolute best. That means managing the track career of the horse, building its fitness up during the year, aiming it for target races and making sure the talent within comes to the fore. Alongside the horse, is the jockey. For the best horses, you want the best rider. The owners want that too. Obviously.

If an owner thinks they're not getting the best from the trainer, they can easily pull their horse and go elsewhere. Most owners don't have just one horse, so when they go, they really tend to up-sticks and can leave a trainer's yard decimated. Therefore the trainers keep the owners happy by making sure the horses reach their peak at the right time and ensuring the best, most capable jockeys are on board.

Now, against this backdrop, Josh had lost his most experienced jump jockey to an illness that most thought he'd never come back from. Yet, despite all the pressures he must have faced from owners, he stuck to his promise and never sought out an experienced jockey to replace me on a permanent basis. Even when he was getting ear ache he stuck to his guns. I was massively fortunate that the stable lads he gave the rides to, Christy Kinane and Richard Rowe were hugely talented and Josh had brought all his horses to peak. The owners wanted winners and I guess while they got them, they backed off pressurising Josh. Not that he would have changed his mind anyway, but I suppose it made things easier. Regardless, what Josh Gifford did for me was wholly remarkable and I'll always be grateful.

As winter moved into spring I was asked by the BBC if I would provide radio commentary for them at the Cheltenham Festival. They'd even pay me. That was nice of them. I'd have probably done it for free. Well, maybe not, but I was more than happy to do it. During the Festival I had the pleasure of covering one of the most satisfying wins I can ever remember on a course.

I've mentioned before a man called Anthony Robinson. He was a racehorse owner, an amateur jockey of considerable skill and one of life's gentlemen. I met him down at Cheltenham and he confided in me something I hadn't been aware of. Anthony had been diagnosed with cancer three years previously and had required major surgery. He'd come through, regained his fitness and applied to have his jockey license renewed by the British Jockey Club, who had turned him down. Not to be put off, he applied to the Irish authorities and got his license back that way, just in time for the Irish Distillers Grand National of 1979. He rode one of his own horses, that little force of nature that was Tied Cottage. A brave and immensely talented battler who almost always made all the running from the front, you'll remember he had seemed about to win the 1979 Cheltenham Gold Cup in the middle of that snow storm, when he fell at the last.

A few weeks after that fall, Anthony mounted up on him and in a gruelling, thrilling and extremely tight race, Tied Cottage won the Irish Grand National by a neck. Typical of his nature, Anthony had insisted no mention of his illness be made. Now Anthony was back and aiming Tied Cottage at another attempt at the Gold Cup. Not that he would be riding it, that job would go to the three times Cup winner, Tommy Carberry.

In the morning, Anthony sought me out on the course and told me his story. He insisted that I shouldn't ever be discouraged in my plan to ride again. It was such a boost to my confidence to hear from someone who had been through the same as me. Later that afternoon I was thrilled and delighted to be able to commentate on the sight of Tied Cottage, after making all the running yet again, clearing the last beautifully and romping home to win by eight lengths. A great victory for a great horse and jockey and owner. How devastating it must have been then, when Tied Cottage was disqualified weeks later on a technicality for trace amounts of contaminants in his feed. Anthony, being such as he was, quietly accepted the judgement, turned up to help present the Gold Cup to Arthur Barrow, the owner of Master Smudge and then treated him to a bottle of champagne in the bar. A great example of treating triumph and disaster in the right way and a mark of the man.

After Cheltenham, the BBC must have thought I'd done okay as they asked me to go up to Aintree and cover the National with them. Obviously, I wasn't going to be riding, so being paid by the Beeb for being there was as good as I could hope for. I got to be interviewed on radio by Derek as we walked round the course, explaining all the fences and the proper lines to take. When we got back to the stands, I managed to pop myself onto the weighing scales. They showed 12st 9lb. I was stunned. In a little over four months I had gotten heavy. I needed to make sure I didn't keep on with that or I'd never get back into a saddle. The National that year was won by Ben Nevis, a 40-1 outsider ridden by an American amateur called Charlie Fenwick. It was a remarkable achievement and one that I intended to emulate the following year.

However, I was still far from being fit and the UK's typical cold and damp weather wasn't doing much to help. I decided, in agreement with Josh, that going back to America might be a good idea. I could still ride out and the weather would be a lot more pleasant. So it was, straight after the National, I flew to join Burly

Cock's yard in South Carolina. As I was packing, I realised I had soft, wispy hairs coming through on my head. I decided I'd leave my wigs at home.

φ

Camden, South Carolina was lovely, the temperature in April was much warmer than England, Burly's training centre was well equipped and the nearby health spa was fantastically kitted out. My routine in the early weeks was rigorous. I would get up early, ride out a number of horses, then head to the spa, workout in the gym on a vast array of equipment, including bikes and treadmills and weights, then a quick sauna, more weights and all of that followed up with a road run. As a fitness program it was excellent, but it relied on riding out good horses and Burly did me proud.

From my arrival he put me on some of the best horses in the States. His faith in me was brilliant and really did spur me on, but I was still getting very tired so much quicker than I ever had, so I was a long way from riding in a race. The main issue for me was the continued lack of feeling in my hands and feet. I'd taken to walking around barefoot, just to encourage a bit of stimulation and maybe increase the circulation. It didn't really do much good and one day Burly sat with me in the garden and looked at me a bit oddly, I asked him was what wrong.

He asked, "Can you feel your feet Bob?"

I assured him I could. Burly pointed to the sole of my foot. I looked down to see a nail sticking half an inch into my heel. He went and got some iodine and pulled it out. After that I went back to wearing shoes.

Generally though, apart from the numbness, I was feeling better, but I certainly wasn't looking back to my best. I knew that because Jonathan Sheppard, the only English trainer down in Camden and a man I knew well, walked right by me one morning. It was only when he'd asked Burly who the new guy was that he came back and apologised to me.

In the last week at Camden, before Burly wanted me to go up to his New York yard, the horse I was riding to exercise fell heavily. It was my first fall since Fury Boy had dislodged me and I jumped up from this one just as I had from that. At least my nerve was undamaged, although the bruises took a while to go down. I'm sure Burly would have had his heart in his mouth, but he didn't really say anything and let me get on with things my way.

About the end of April, I travelled north and stayed with Tommy Skiffington. Each day I'd exercise at least six horses around the famous Belmont track, home to the Belmont Stakes, part of America's famous Triple Crown. Between the racing and the continued exercising I had dropped more than a stone from my weight on the Aintree scales. I was feeling slimmer and stronger. My muscle definition was returning, albeit slowly and at last, my hair was showing marked signs of recovery. I think, deep down, this may have pleased me more than all the rest of the improvements. After staying with Tommy, I moved up to Unionville in Pennsylvania, Burly's main training facility. I spent another week there riding for him and making use of the exercise facilities and the tennis courts. All in all things were progressing really, really well. Except for my feet. And my hands.

Occasionally when running, I'd fall over because I quite literally couldn't feel my feet on the ground. I'd also drop things because I had little feeling in my fingers. Despite these minor issues, Burly suggested that I might be able to ride in a proper race within a month or two. That was a huge boost and one I needed as I headed back home to England for another set of hospital tests.

The results were as good as before. Everything was looking good. The doctors were a bit shocked, if I'm honest. They hadn't expected me to be as well as I was. They were even more surprised when I mentioned that I might be race riding soon.

I spent two weeks at home and rode out for Paul Cole again most days, because I couldn't let things lapse, even for a short while. On one notable day, I rode out for Josh. Then I had a couple of phone calls that definitely told me I was on my way back.

The first was from Jim Old who asked me if I would ride Joint Venture at Newton Abbott on the 21st May. Swiftly followed by a call from Jonathan Sheppard over in America, asking me if I'd take a phenomenal opportunity on a top-class chaser, Martie's Anger in a $25,000 race at Hard Scuffle on the 24th May. That horse had a real chance and the jockey's share of the prize money would be about $2,500. That was quite a pay packet after the amount of time I'd been out of work. More significant was that I'd been offered my first two professional rides since coming back. I was delighted.

I turned both of them down.

Joint Venture was a good horse with a good chance, but I knew in myself that I was still at least a week or two away from being fit enough and added to that, I wanted my first race in England to be on a horse trained by Josh. Jim Old was generous enough to understand. The American option was easier. The horse was too good a chance in a major race with significant prize money. I couldn't be making my debut in something like that. It wouldn't have been fair to the horse, the owners, Jonathan or myself. Like Jim, Jonathan understood. As it was, Joint Venture finished a disappointing third and Martie's Anger romped home a worthy winner.

Before I went back to the States, I was approached by the Sunday People newspaper for an interview. At first I refused, but it was the doctors at the Royal Marsden who convinced me that I should do it. They thought it would send a positive message to the other patients on the cancer wards. I could hardly say no after that. When the article came out, I started getting a lot of letters congratulating me and thanking me. Some of the most inspiring were from patients on cancer wards who said they had taken hope from my story. I was really chuffed and I made sure I answered every single letter personally. It was something that I made sure I did every time I got a letter like that and still do, although it's mostly emails nowadays. I'd often get letters from family members asking if I could send a few words of encouragement, which I always did. I cannot express the pleasure it gave me when, a year or so later, I'd hear back directly from the person telling me that they'd recovered and how they were getting their lives back together.

I returned to America and on the 30th May Jonathan Sheppard asked me to ride a horse called Ripon in a race at Fairhill the next day. Back at the start of my career I'd have said, 'yes please', but riding a comeback race on a horse who had, on its first two outings, fallen quite heavily was not on my immediate list of things to do. I dissuaded Jonathan from running him and tootled off to have a meal with some friends. When I got back to my digs, Jonathan was there waiting for me.

"Will you ride Double Reefed then?"

"When?"

"Tomorrow, at Fairhill."

"But that's entered in a flat race isn't it?"

"Yes. No chance of falling."

"It's doubtful I'll make the weight."

"You'll only be a few pounds over. I'll take the chance. Will you?"

"I guess so."

So that was it. My comeback would be in an American flat race.

I woke early, rode out a few horses and then set off with Jonathan. Interestingly, Fairhill isn't your normal American oval dirt track. It's a grass country course, almost the same as an English National Hunt course, so I was in fairly familiar surroundings. As for Double Reefed, apparently he'd been a good flat prospect earlier in his career but had gone off the boil. Jonathan was considering putting him up over hurdles, but in a last effort to get him going again he thought he'd try him out on the Fairhill grass. What Jonathan didn't know was that I'd never ridden in a flat race in my life. He discovered it in the car on the way there, but he stuck with me.

I weighed out five pounds over at 11st 6lb and then tried to decipher the confusing US form guide to figure out who the other riders and horses were. It seemed Double Reefed, despite its recent form, was going to go off as favourite. I wondered at the sanity of that, although I'd ridden the horse on exercise runs back at the yard and knew he had quite a turn of speed.

One year and twenty days after Fury Boy kicked me in the nuts, I lined up at the start of my comeback race. The field came under starter's orders and then, we were off. I held Double Reefed at the back and nestled into the inside rail approaching the first of the tight left-hand bends on the one mile and 5/16 distance. The rest of the runners drifted a bit wide and gave me a clear run, so I took the shortest way round, but didn't press forward. We stuck to last place and I held him in his rhythm until the last half mile. Then we started to pick our way through on the inside rail. At the final bend, about three furlongs out, I couldn't believe that the leaders all drifted wide again. I asked a little more of Double Reefed and he delivered. The strangest thought came into my head with about two furlongs to go, 'I'm going to win this!'

Frankly, right up until then I hadn't considered that as even a remote possibility. I had thought it was a chance to test myself and see how far I had come and how far I still had to go in terms of fitness. Now, sitting in third place and knowing, just knowing that I could take the two horses in front at any time, I started to think like a proper jockey again. I waited until the final furlong marker and then I pushed him forward. Blow me if he didn't try and duck in behind the backsides of the two in front. 'Not a chance,' I thought and gave him a single hard smack. He immediately picked up and surged into the lead. We kept accelerating and won it easily. I was puffed, but not as bad as I'd thought I would be and it didn't matter because I'd won. I was well chuffed. I was back. I was a jockey… and a flat one to boot!

I got quite the reception on my return to the changing room as the rest of the jockeys knew what I was coming back from. To show their congratulations they did that peculiar American thing of throwing a few buckets of cold water over me! I got dried and changed and then, as best I could, I slipped away for a while. In fact I wandered around the now quiet Fairhill for about an hour. I needed some time on my own to process what had happened. I don't just mean the race, I mean all of it. The diagnosis, the treatment, the striving to get back and then, yes, the race. The fact I had won on my first race back was overwhelming. I can remember wanting to laugh and cry and shout and yell and be very quiet all at once. It was intense.

Eventually I came back and got led off to a bar, followed by a few more drinks, followed by going to a dance and then more drinks. I allegedly, although it is all a bit hazy, rang Mary and a few other friends to let them know what had happened. At 4am we called it quits. At 6am, for the first time in all his many, many years of training, Burly had to cancel his planned day because there wasn't one of us fit to ride a horse to exercise. He sent us all back to bed and let the horses stay in their stables. A memorable couple of days indeed.

Because there is very little in the way of jump racing in America during June, most of the rest of my time was spent exercising horses and myself. That said, I did get one more ride on Ripon at Monmouth Park in which we finished third. Then it was time to go back home for the next set of follow-up tests.

The doctors were, without exaggeration, baffled at how well my lungs had recovered. As I waited for the final results, I went up to the adult cancer ward to say thanks to Carol, Jenny, Nicky and all the other nurses. I also wanted to walk in there and show the rest of the patients that this was doable. You could come back, you could recover, you could beat this damned thing.

I was aware that many who do survive do not want to go anywhere near the ward again. It feels like a bad place to return to, full of dark memories. But I figured that had a survivor come to see me when I was in there, it would have been a good experience. I knew it would have made a big difference to me, so I decided to be that person. If it gave hope in a small way to just one person, then it was worth it.

Afterwards, because the docs were so pleased with all my results, I asked if they could delay my next check-up so that I could have a longer stay back in the States. They readily agreed and after a quick three-day trip to Ireland to stay with Tommy Stack and his wife Liz, I set off to what I hoped would be renewed glory.

It wasn't.

φ

I knew my first win at Fairhill had been when I wasn't fully fit. I reckon I'd been maybe eighty-five percent, so I threw myself back into training hard. Of course I had the renewed and constant issue of my weight to deal with and sometimes both Burly and Jonathan would come along and tell me to ease off all the dieting as it wasn't good for me.

Throughout July I couldn't catch a cold let alone many rides and certainly no winners and then in the August we moved with the rest of the circuit up to the beautiful Saratoga. I got to ride Double Reefed again, but this time over fences. We won again. I did like that horse and switching him to fences was the smart move by Jonathan as a year or so later he would go on to be a champion steeplechaser. I liked him especially on that day at Saratoga as my share of the prize money was $1,600. In a standard novice chase, that was ridiculous money compared to the paltry sums in Britain. I was delighted and then, a couple of days later, I was bereft.

I got word that Anthony Robinson had passed away. I was so, so sorry to hear that. He'd put up such a good fight, been cleared of the cancer once and looked to be well on the way to a full life again. He deserved better. To be honest, I was shattered and not a little frightened. I suppose I wondered that if it could come back in Anthony…

From when I had the disease right up to the present day, every time someone dies of cancer it frightens me not a little, but the loss of Anthony was a very personal thing. It affected me then and to some extent, still affects me now, on a much deeper level than I would care to admit. He was forty-three.

A few weeks later, the Sunday Times sent Brough Scott and a photographer called Gerry Cranham over to do a piece on me. We had a great old time water skiing and swimming and jet skiing, oh and taking in some of the racing at Saratoga too. I was okay with them doing a press piece on me because Brough had been such a stalwart supporter when I'd been in the hospital. Gerry too had been very kind and sent a great photo of me winning at Kempton in the hope of buoying me up. It had worked well. I still have that picture.

When the piece came out it was really good. It described my journey, starting in the depths of despair in the ward, when Brough would visit and, now he was able to admit it, go along with my ludicrous desire to be a jockey again just to show solidarity. He wrote that he would leave the ward and feel thoroughly depressed driving home in his car and how, each time he said goodbye, he thought it would be the last. The article ended with me, eight months later, out in America, riding winners, reclaiming my fitness, my health restored and having a grand old time surrounded by a bevy of beautiful women. The main thing that surprised both Brough and Gerry was how many horses I would ride out to exercise each day. They both thought that eight was remarkable. I had to tell them eight was a light day. On occasion I would saddle up sixteen, thanks to 'Bubba', Burly's head groom who would get me lots of spare rides with all the nearby yards. He was a smashing guy, looked the spitting image of Muhammad Ali and used to call me, 'Big Bob' because I was so much bigger than all the other jockeys. We would be up and about a lot earlier than anyone else and certainly always ahead of the other yards. One day I noticed we were short on some tack. I asked Bubba where the nearest saddlers was.

He gave me an all-knowing look. "What do we need to go to the saddlers for Big Bob?"

I explained why and he simply said, "Leave it with me, we don't need to be going to any saddlers. You'll see in the morning."

Sure enough, next day the tack room was full of what we wanted. I decided I probably didn't need to ask how this magic had happened.

There's no doubt in my mind that exercising all the extra rides Bubba found allowed me to reclaim my fitness so much more quickly. I definitely came back fitter and stronger after the cancer than I had been before.

That month in Saratoga was not only good for me physically. The racing season in America goes round in a circuit and in that summer month at Saratoga there was a real sense of the holiday spirit. Practically every evening there would be a concert on, with such an eclectic mix of big bands over the month, from the Beach Boys through to the Philadelphia Philharmonic Orchestra. I'm not that into classical music but the Philharmonic played modern hits and it was brilliant. All the yard would go along, pay our $5 and sit with a big, huge in fact, bucket of fried chicken. Then we'd go to bed and get up next morning to ride work again.

During our occasional full days off a bunch of us jockeys would either mess around on jet skis at Lake George or, occasionally, we'd head up to a ski resort in nearby Vermont. Of course, being summer there wasn't much snow about, but this place had an Alpine Slide, which is basically a huge fibreglass slide all the way down the mountain. Imagine a downhill twisting, curving bobsleigh run, but made out of hard plastic. You went down it on a little sledge, like a tray on wheels, lying flat and using your feet as brakes. It was okay, but a dozen jockeys reckoned it was pretty boring and probably not as fast as it could have been. I decided, as the token 'Mad Englishman', that if all twelve of us got on a little sledge each and lined up behind one another like a big train, we'd be bound to go faster. There was surely some scientific principle that could be applied, although I remember thinking later I should probably have paid more attention in those physics classes at school. However, not to be undone by a lack of theory with regard to 'Bob's Law of Physics' we went for the practical test. Things were looking good and then about a third of the way down, when our speed had really built up, we swept round a long left-hand bend and then at the next right-hander we all went straight on. The sledges left the track, carried by our momentum up and over the side and into a Vermont sky.

Oh, it was carnage. We were sprawled over half a mountainside, bruised and battered and bloodied. Any that had been unfortunate enough to land back on the fibreglass were burnt to ribbons. Their clothes were shredded and they had big welts on their skin. It was horrendous and some of the best fun we ever had.

You couldn't help but laugh as this battered dozen of jockeys, suffering from more bruises than we'd ever have gotten in a race, gingerly picked ourselves up. I decided not to announce that at least 'Bob's Law' had been proven true. We'd certainly gone faster.

That was a fantastic time in my life and you could be forgiven for wondering why I came back at all. The answer is simple really. There wasn't enough jump racing in the States and more than that, I wanted to make it at home again, on the biggest and best National Hunt courses, including that dream of Aldaniti at Aintree. That and Josh had promised that he would keep my job open for me.

I had of course been in constant touch with him whilst I was out in the States and he'd kept me informed of when he was putting his runners back onto the track, but it was likely to be nearer the end of August, so I stayed put for a while longer. Great as it was, I wasn't getting many rides and apart from Double Reefed, no winners. My last week at Saratoga was particularly annoying.

I had a ride on a horse and approaching the finish it was obvious we couldn't win. I put my whip hand down and rode him out to finish second. The stewards fined me $200 for failing to ride the horse to achieve the best possible placing. It was nonsense and I was really annoyed. I might not have been fully fit but I'm damned if I stopped riding properly at any time. That's almost thirty years ago now and it still rankles me. Then, on the day I was due to fly home, I had my last ride on Café Prince, one of the best chasers in the US and twice winner of the Colonial Cup. You couldn't have told any of that from the way he went about his business that day. Jumping like a novice he absolutely buried me into hard ground. I had to convince the course doctor I hadn't been knocked out just so he would let me fly. I felt awful, concussed, battered, with a black eye and a cut to my nose, I looked like some weird street thug on board the plane. Add to that I was sick a fair few times in the air and with a good measure of jet lag my triumphant homecoming was anything but. However, America had served her purpose. I was well on my way to fulfilling the dream that I had set. It was the last week in August and the Grand National was seven months and a few days away.

Now the real hard work began.

φ

Val and Pete from the Hungerford Squash Club stepped straight back in to help me on my arrival home. Running, weight training and physio massage would restore my physical presence. Josh and his offer of the ride on Roadhead at Stratford on the 30th August would restore my spirit.

The August meeting at Stratford is hardly the normal cause for a huge press turnout, but that day was the exception. I was greeted by a copy of the Sporting Life with a banner headline say-ing 'Hail Champion the Wonder Horseman' with an accompanying big photo and a warm welcome back message. I was chuffed, but also bemused. This wasn't Fairhill where hardly anyone really knew who I was, this was National Hunt and it seemed half the UK press were here to cover it. Add to that poor Roadhead, who I had won many a race on previously, was top weight and although I had always liked him and he was a safe jumper, I never figured he would stay much past two and a half miles. The City of Coventry Handicap Chase at Stratford was another quarter mile further. All in all, I was nervous, although all the other jockeys made me feel that I was properly 'back home' and the banter relaxed me a bit.

Alas, this was to be no Double Reefed return. We had a good run, held the lead a couple of times, but the extra trip and huge top weight meant we could only finish a close, and respectable, fourth. Probably not what the press had wanted, but it had been painless, the owners were happy and Josh was delighted. I was relieved that I hadn't made a fool of myself on my return and completely content with the way I had ridden. But three days later at Plumpton, it was a different matter altogether. I was on one of Josh's called Toureen who was mediocre at best and at his last outing had finished tailed off last. The fact he was second favourite here was due to a bit of sympathy money for me. Off we went and unsurprisingly Toureen didn't jump well, weakened in the closing stages and finished last. But what had shocked me was the way I had dropped my reins when Toureen had gone through the top of one of the fences.

To explain, you have to know that most jockeys when taking a jump at race speed will slip the reins to the end of the buckle. It gives the horse's head a freedom of movement so that if it pecks on landing you're not dragged out of the saddle and ejected into the ground. I slipped them, but then I dropped them completely. I man-aged to get them back but the problem was I still couldn't feel my hands properly. They were nearly always numb or occasionally had intense pins and needles. I contacted the hospital and the best Doc-tor Jane could tell me was that it was another side-effect of chemo and would improve as time went on. That wasn't great news, but the season was about to take a much worse turn.

The Jockey Club, in the run up to the winter of 1980, issued an order that all horses were to be given an anti-flu jab. Nobody argued against the correctness of the order, but the timing was all wrong. As Josh said, "We should have had two year's notice, or at the very least it should have been administered at the start of the summer break so they could have recovered. As it was, all my horses were knocked sideways for months."

September was therefore, lean in the extreme and I took myself and a girlfriend on a short break to Ireland. Whilst there I picked up a couple of rides in Galway but they didn't amount to much. The hospitality and company was as usual, 'great craic' as the Irish would say and like most breaks to that nation, I really needed a holiday to recover once I'd come home, but there was to be no time. Josh had decided to run a horse called Physicist at Fontwell on the 23rd September. It was one of the few in the yard that hadn't been given the flu jab because he wouldn't be running later in the season, so he was still fresh and up for it.

By now the press interest in me had slackened off a bit, but they were still writing stories about my comeback and I knew they were still watching out for me, so I was still nervous. If anything, not winning had put a lot more pressure on me. I said earlier, this whole sports person's confidence is a fragile thing. Like the striker on a barren run of form, with no goals and a feeling like they'd smash it over the bar from less than six yards. It all adds up to put a mental tax on you. Like part of your attention is distracted by the need to have a result, and without total concentration you can't get the result. It makes you want to scream. Or, in my case at Fontwell, pace around and around the weighing room like a caged tiger.

Then it was time and I joined Josh in the paddock. He gave me his last instructions, "Right Bob, don't forget that he's short of work, so look after him. If you do get into a finish only hit him the once. He's far from fully wound up and I don't want him having a hard race."

There was a field of six and we set off for what would be three full circuits of the tight figure-of-eight Fontwell track. The only real risk to Physicist was Bold Saint, but I reckoned he wouldn't have the legs for the three and a quarter miles. As we came into the final circuit, I eased Physicist a little to give him a breather, jumped the next two fences, took a marginal lead from the early pacesetters and looked to my right to see Bold Saint come cruising past me going easily. So much for my theory about him not having the legs for it. I checked over my shoulder and the rest of the field were slipping backwards, so I figured a comfortable second was on the cards, but over the third from home it was obvious that Bold Saint wasn't increasing his lead. I gave Physicist a bit of a squeeze and he pinged the fence, gaining a length. Then I relaxed him a bit, gave him another breather, then rode him into the second last. Another length gained. The same on the run up to the last, just keeping the momentum going then riding for the fence. Another length and by now we were within touching distance. Fontwell's finish is a step uphill and all the way up it Bold Saint maintained his advantage, but we were closing and closing and closing. I admit, I may have forgotten Josh's instructions and given Physicist a fair few reminders to keep him moving, but in the last twenty strides we edged past Bold Saint and won by half a length.

I can remember it being warm and bright and sunny and the crowd being a good size for Fontwell, though what I remember most was the deafening noise of cheering and applause. It was very humbling as I came into the winner's circle and dismounted. Then a woman who seemed very pleased for me came up and gave me a great kiss. It was only fair to return it.

This happened often and women would follow the jockeys around. It's like any sporting profession, you have your fan clubs and women like to follow fit men. We certainly never did anything untoward and most of us were very careful about the ladies we dated. It's very sad to see so many 'celebrities' from back in those days having appeared to have abused their position and their fame. Of course we loved the attention and we all enjoyed how flattering it was, but I know I would certainly never have done anything wrong and neither would any of my friends.

Back in the 1960s it had been all the go as well. In fact Brough Scott wrote about the time when he was a young apprentice and the jockeys, Josh Gifford (yes, my Guv'nor Josh) and Terry Biddlecombe would take him out. Neither Josh nor Terry were retiring wall-flower types. Brough remembered, '...that spending one evening on the lash with Josh and Terry would fix most people. How they would do it week after week only their livers could tell.'

It really was quite the cavalier lifestyle, going out after racing, staying up most of the night, then hitting the sauna or Turkish baths to lose all the excess weight the next day. I was just lucky that I didn't share the fairly heavy drinking most of the guys did. The reality is, it was a very different time for jump racing. There were no breathalysers or tests done before we raced the next day, so we could get away with it.

I know that Derek Thompson can attest to the phenomenon of the fans because he caught me on one occasion having a bit of a kiss and a cuddle between races with three different girls.

Honestly, I was never, ever one for trying chat up lines or being Mr Cool. Far from it. I was the shy and honest one, but that seemed to be just the thing some of the women were looking for, so who was I to argue? I was single, young and fit. Jockey's weren't rich, but we weren't broke either. The lads would joke with me about getting kitted up early and riding round the paddock just to see if we had any admirers watching. There'd always be a few and I'd give them a little smile to let them know I'd seen them. If I didn't have a bad fall then I knew I'd probably have a date that evening.

Physicist was my first winner in England for nearly seventeen months and I was really pleased that my first comeback winner had been on a horse Josh had trained. It somehow seemed fitting and proper. I didn't realise until later that it was Josh's 500th winner since he became a trainer. Given the two events, I think I recall a little celebration that night.

Three or so days later and I was at Stratford in a televised meeting. Once more the cameras seemed to follow me around more than normal and Lord Oaksey, who was commentating, spent quite a while describing my comeback win and how, today, I was on Kindly Night in the opening novice chase. I was quietly confident and we set off on a slippy surface that was nearly the undoing of us at the first. Struggling over it we continued, although detached from the rest of the field but that wasn't to matter as at the second, Kindly Night went straight into the open ditch, flipped a complete somersault and fired me out of the saddle. The nation's television viewers were able to see me bounced into the air like a trapeze art- ist. I don't think I have ever gone higher in a fall. Frankie Dettori had nothing on me! Thankfully, I landed on my nose and hand and more importantly, Kindly Night landed beside me rather than on me. I was just winded but it took me a while to lie there and get my breath back. Then, when I figured out there was nothing wrong with me, I got up.

Annoyingly, after the last televised race, I rode Roadhead in the Klampenborg Chase and won easily, but there was no one there to record it for posterity. The following Saturday however, in front of the BBC cameras I had my first televised win since coming back. Then in the next race, just to make sure I didn't get carried away with myself, I was ploughed into the ground by a horse called Right Mingle. Thankfully, both it and the Kindly Night fall had been heavy yet I'd come through them alright. It's a testament to the idiocy of the average jump jockey that we think being thumped into the ground and not having anything but bruises all over us, is a good thing.

The season progressed and I had a few more winners in the October, but by now I was getting a bit fed up with all of the press interest. They were still going on and on about how remarkable it was that I had come back, like I was some sort of Lazarus figure. I'd given the earlier press interviews at the encouragement of the doctors at the Royal Marsden and the letters I was still getting from other cancer patients, or their friends and family were proof that it had been the right thing to do, but now I just wanted to move on. I also didn't know why the press and everyone else seemed so surprised. It wasn't like I hadn't told everyone that would listen that I'd comeback to be a jockey again.

All in all I thought I was doing okay, but my weight was giving me a bit of concern. Then it started giving me a lot of concern. Doctor Jane told me it was likely, that as a side-effect of the chemo, I might find myself heavier than I had been before the treatment. Yet again, that mattered little to most survivors, but to me... well you get the picture. In mid-October I realised that my natural weight was settling at 12st 7lbs. I would never get a ride in National Hunt at that weight. All of the starving and wasting and sweating and saunas in my past had, it turned out, been child's play compared to what I was going to need to do. But there would be no pills this time. I'd had enough of drugs. It meant that all the sweeties and cakes and other rubbish I used to keep at home went in the bin and I started paying proper attention to what I ate and drank.

I spoke to Josh, and he told me that if I could get down to 10st 10lb then he'd be okay with it. The trouble is that jockeys aren't boxers. We don't get to strip to our underwear to get weighed. We need to be wearing and carrying everything that is going on the horse, so that includes our clothes, our saddle, the breastplates, girths, stirrups and anything else, including blinkers or hoods. That all added up to sometimes as much as 5lbs, which meant to get to Josh's desired weight I'd be at about 10½st, roughly what I was before the chemo. It was hard going, but interestingly I found it a struggle that I could cope with. Yes it meant no more parties celebrating winners, yes it meant hours and hours in horrendously hot saunas, yes it meant even more exercising and working out, yes, it required an even harsher discipline, but it was a battle against something I could see and understand. That and the fact I hadn't come this far for my weight to stop me riding. Anyway, I'm nothing if not stubborn, so by constant and continuous effort, I got it under control. What I had no control over was what almost made me jack the whole thing in.

φ

Football teams that aren't doing well sack the manager as a first move. Racehorse owners blame the jockey. It's that simple and it doesn't take too much to start the rot. In fact, it can go from good to bad very quickly. Basically, Josh's horses were doing atrociously due to the flu jab and if I am being brutally honest, I was trying too hard.

The problems set in at Kempton on the 18th October when Roadhead slipped going into the third in the Charisma Records Gold Cup. The horse lost its confidence and barely made it round to finish almost last. Now I had won on Roadhead seven times previously, but the owners told Josh in no uncertain terms they wanted Richard Rowe on him next time out.

My next ride was on Fredo, a young promising novice making his debut over fences. Except he didn't get over the first. Then Earthstopper at Cheltenham lost by a short-head, then Fredo again at Ascot, who managed to clear the obstacles this time but finished in a poor fifth. Things were not going well.

I managed a brief positive on Glamour Show on the last day of October at Huntingdon in the Sydney Banks Hurdle, but only just in a photo finish and the owners weren't convinced, so I lost the ride on him for the next time out as well. The next day, Socks and I parted company at the fifth and his owner, Douglas Bunn decided that as Richard Rowe had ridden and won on Socks four times while I'd been ill, he'd go back to him. Fair enough.

The only bright spot was that Carol, the sister from the cancer ward had come to see me ride that day. She was really worried when I got carted back from the fifth in the rear of the course ambulance, but I was fine. Just a bit bruised. She said that I'd looked fantastic on the horse, but she thought I was crazy to have fought so hard to survive cancer just to come back to a sport that could, quite literally, kill me. Yeah, maybe. I only knew that my lack of form was certainly trying my spirit.

On the 5th November, even Josh got annoyed at me. I had the ride on Snow Flyer and was given specific instructions in the paddock, within earshot of the owners.

"He's a brilliant horse, Bob but he's had his leg problems, so settle in behind the rest, take it steady and conserve him for the finish. His welfare comes first, understand?"

"Yes."

It was soon evident Snow Flyer hadn't listened in to the conversation when, at the first, he gave a breath-taking leap and went in to the lead. A place we stayed, galloping along and leaping freely until the eleventh when we galloped straight through it and I was dumped. On my return the owners were speechless and Josh, far from happy. I tried to explain that I hadn't deliberately disobeyed the orders and that Snow Flyer, seeing daylight around him had taken a flyer, much like his name. There was nothing I, nor any other jockey, could have done.

Half an hour later, my day got worse. Riding Moonlight Express, he sprawled at the fifth and that was that chance gone. Even my one winner that afternoon, on Lumen in a hurdle race, was an anti-climax. We were halfway up the finishing straight, going easy with a distance back to the rest, when a horse called Palace Dan came back at us strongly. It was very close, but I just held on to take it in a photo finish. However, the punters in the stands, the horse's owner, Peter Hopkins and Josh all thought I had been much too casual in the run in. In my defence, I had ridden Lumen before and I had the distinct impression that he hated the whip. Possibly he'd been given too much of it when as a younger horse he'd raced on the flat, so I only rode him hand and heels. It had worked, but the people that mattered were not happy.

The next Saturday, with three meetings on, I didn't have one ride.

I moped about and was acutely aware of what could happen. Josh's horses were out of sorts. I was out of form. Owners had started pulling their rides from me and that meant I had less rides to prove everyone wrong. Because of that, other trainers weren't likely to offer me a ride and so a vicious circle had begun. I wondered if it was all worth it.

However, on the Monday I got up and went back to Findon to ride out for Josh. There was a TV company there to do a pre-arranged feature on me and thankfully they followed me up to

Fontwell to see me win a novice chase on Ta Jette. I also heard Josh telling them he still supported me as his stable jockey. I took a boost from the day. Just as well. I was going to need it.

For the rest of November I had a few opportunities but couldn't ride a winner. The bitter icing on that particular cake was that Richard Rowe, who had done so well in the season when I was out had been requested by the owners to take the rides on Earth-stopper and Glamour Show. He duly won on them both.

I knew I was trying too hard. Josh knew it too and had taken to giving me a lot more instructions than he had in the past, but he was always supportive, never condemning, so that was a huge bonus, but things were definitely far from ideal. To add to the worry and my sleepless nights, the next set of hospital tests were coming up on the 27th. Once more though, the worrying was for nowt. I was still cancer-free. I should have been ecstatic for the rest of my life. As it was, I was happy for about two days.

Then I was told that I had lost the ride on Fredo. I'm not quite sure why that particular news hit me as hard as it did, but I sunk into what I can now see was depression. I thought there was no point in going on. Even my new girlfriend, Jo, couldn't snap me out of it. I was fed up with all of it. I knew racing was a hard game and I knew Josh's owners had supported me all through my illness, but now, when I was trying to make good my comeback, their patience had worn thin. It seemed to me that I only had two options. One was to go to the States and possibly become a trainer, the other was to stay and fight for my career as a jockey. I wasn't sure there was any fight left in me. If I left Josh's yard and looked for owners and trainers who would give me a go, I was likely to be massively disappointed.

With my future not decided as yet, I travelled to Fontwell on the 3rd December to ride Right Mingle again. First though I would have a ride in a novice chase on a good young horse called Topseed. We were going well when we fell on the flat between fences. He just flipped out from underneath me travelling round the top bend. I was knocked hard and returned to the weighing room obviously concussed and with a hell of a limp. The course doctor told me I wouldn't be riding again that day. Half an hour later I watched from the stands as Richard stood in for me and rode Right Mingle to the easiest of victories.

By the 13th December I was thinking that I'd probably call it quits. But first I had to go to Ascot. I'd not had a winner in five weeks and my first ride that day, Pillager didn't change the statistic. The next race was the SGB Chase in which a small field of four contained Venture to Cognac, probably the best young chaser in Britain. Sadly, I wasn't on him. Neither was I on one of the other two horses who were pretty handy. Instead I was on Henry Bishop.

We set off, me feeling pretty shabby with life and all it was throwing at me. Not unsurprisingly we were last all the way round and going into the final mile, when all of a sudden I realised... Henry Bishop was travelling strongly. It's like someone turned me back on. I jumped the fourth last and closed to within a length of Venture to Cognac, then took the lead three out. Working our way up Ascot's long hill I opened a six length advantage which I kept over the second last. Then I could feel Henry Bishop weakening, but no one was closing us down significantly so I concentrated on safely getting over the last. Once over I could sense Venture to Cognac mounting an effort but I drove home hard and we won by two lengths. Of all the races I have ever won, the sense of relief from that one was the biggest. Whatever the owners or the press or the punters thought, I could still be a proper winning jockey and bring a horse home.

I was bouncing and it couldn't have come at a better time for about half an hour later I was reunited with an old favourite of mine, the magnificent Kybo, who I'd come so close to Champion Hurdle success on. Since then, during my illness, he'd been swapped to fences and won two of his three starts with Richard on board, before a spot of leg trouble had convinced Josh to pull him out of training. This was his return to the track after a thirteen month layoff and although he was unbeaten over five starts at Ascot, today in the Frogmore Chase, it was highly unlikely that run would continue. He was carrying a heavy handicap weight due to previous successes, the distance was short of his best and he needed one run at least to get back into top form. Josh told me in no uncertain terms to look after the horse and just enjoy myself. For my part,

I planned to settle at the back, use Kybo's amazing speed to pick off the rest of the field one by one and pull him up as soon as he laboured.

Off we went and put the plan into action. A comfortable romp round the first half mile at the rear of the field of ten, about twenty-five lengths off the leader. Then we were coming down the hill, heading for the famous Swinley Bottom and at each of the fences on that hill we put in a good jump and passed a few of the lesser horses. Turning at the foot of the hill for that long run home I wondered if good old Kybo could surprise everyone, including me. Three from home and we were into fourth but then I felt him lose his action and my instant thought was that he'd gone lame. I made to pull him up, but he had just decided to change his leg and once he'd sorted himself out he went after the leaders with a renewed vigour. I took a moment to make sure he was fine and then let him get on with it. We were fractionally headed by Dramatist, a useful chaser in his own right going into the last fence, but Kybo sailed over it, gained at least half a length in the air and we sprinted to the post for the win. As soon as we were past the post I thought I could feel him unsound again so I hopped off him immediately. Thankfully he was fine and I felt elated. In the space of two races all the negative thoughts and feelings of despair lifted. Although I was slightly embarrassed at the Sporting Life headline on the Monday which praised me again as 'Champion the Wonder Jockey'. These headline writers needed a new angle. As for me, I actually did feel wonderful, but I wasn't about to tell a reporter that. It's a long time ago now, yet I can still point to that day at Ascot for saving my career. I was very close to jacking it all in when Henry Bishop and Kybo restored my faith in myself.

I met up that evening with a lovely young lady, Sarah Wickins, whom I dropped off at the pub before nipping home briefly. On my way back it seemed my bad luck with cars hadn't run its course as I skidded on a patch of mud and the car took off, went straight over a fence and landed on its roof in a ploughed field. I trudged to the pub and told Sarah. Now my memory is a bit hazy how the rest of it came about, but her Dad owned British Car Auctions and after hearing of my news they offered to sponsor me! I don't know what happened with Sarah, but I do know I had a lovely Mercedes to drive around in for a year!

Although Henry Bishop and Kybo had helped me regain my confidence, the winners certainly didn't keep coming as regularly as before. Josh was convinced that most of the problem was down to the flu jab. His veterinarian bills for the yard had quadrupled and he was really quite desperate for an upturn in the condition of the horses.

In the meantime he allowed me to go off on the following Saturday and take a few rides for other trainers. For the second successive week in front of television cameras I rode two winners. It gave me another huge boost and a magnum of champagne from the Racing Information Bureau. It also, in a roundabout way, sent a signal to those owners of Josh's who had been having doubts about me.

Christmas was the norm for me as a jump jockey. Eat little while everyone else eats as much as they can, but it was great to spend it down with Mary, Richard and the kids. My parents were also there so it was great family day, even if I had to go off to a sauna that night in preparation for the big Boxing Day meetings.

The pounds lost in sweat were rewarded by a winner at Huntingdon and then at Cheltenham on New Year's Eve, I had the stereotypical jump jockey's day. A heavy fall in a hurdle race, bumped and bruised but otherwise okay, back to the weighing room, get changed for the next ride, a chase on Kybo, win, lift almost £500 in prize money, have an interview on TV with Julian Wilson, then get buried at the sixth in the next race, dislocate thumb, ignore it, drive home, go to sauna and sweat some more.

The following day's significance wasn't lost on me. It was a year since the end of my last chemo session. I drove to Leicester and had the sixteenth winner of the season on Right Mingle. The journey back to being a jockey hadn't been easy, far from it, but none of that mattered. Racing was what I wanted to do. In reality, it was all of me and anyway, I had a dream to fulfil.

φ

On the 2nd January I arrived at Newbury to discover that I had been awarded the Amoco National Hunt Jockey of the Month for December. Quite surreal given that for the first thirteen days of that month I had almost been ready to quit, but I knew it was in recognition of the successive Saturday doubles and how good Kybo had made me look. The prize was one hundred gallons of petrol (I wish someone would give me that now) and an inscribed whip. It was really nice and I was very chuffed. In fact, up until then and for a long, long time afterwards, that award was the most special to me. It somehow was a recognition to Carol, Jenny, Josh and Mary and all the others that had stuck by me.

Of course, racing being racing, I couldn't be feeling good for too long, so in the first race I fell heavily at an open ditch and the horse, Another Duke, kicked me in the head and rolled over my legs. It took quite a while for me to be convinced that I couldn't ride in the next, but eventually I was feeling so ill and concussed that I submitted. Good job really as the horse I was meant to ride fell with a real crunch at the same open ditch.

After another sauna and a massage from Val, I was back riding the next day. Now you can begin to see how we definitely abused the lack of tight medical controls. I'm glad to say that there is little chance of anything like that occurring today. Back then, it was simply the norm. Wins would be followed by falls and I dislocated the same thumb a couple of times more. Val kept popping it back and I kept riding. Numb hands or not, I could feel that thumb. By the 17th January the month had averaged out to be not too bad at all, but that Saturday at Ascot was to be a terrible, heart-breaking day.

I had rides on two horses, both of whom I knew and one of whom I thought was incredible. The first race on Right Mingle didn't end well as he dumped me off and galloped away to complete the course riderless. The next ride was on my great companion Kybo, in the Jock Scott Handicap Chase.

Going well as usual, Kybo slipped on landing at the water jump, almost did the splits but just about managed to recover, although we were a long way off the running. I decided to pull him up, but he seemed to get back into his stride, much as he had on our last win at Ascot, so I let him jump over a couple more fences on the way back, just to restore his confidence. Kybo went over them like his old self, with no problems at all and I began to pull him up at the entrance to the finishing straight. As he slowed, his near-hind leg shattered just above the hock.

The suddenness of it made him collapse and he threw me clear over the running rail. Then he struggled back up and limped across to the adjacent hurdling track before collapsing again. The course vet had no choice but to swiftly and painlessly euthanise him.

I knew what had happened and ran to Kybo, but he was gone. I took off the saddle and bridle and gave him a farewell pat on the neck, before turning to see Josh running toward me. Neither of us could speak. I walked off towards the stands feeling tragic. It always seems to be the good ones that go far too soon. All of us that knew and worked with him were inconsolable. He'd been such a brave horse and I can say, much as I loved Aldaniti, Kybo was the best I ever rode. I wish so much that I'd pulled him up immediately, but the racecourse vet said it would have made no difference. He said the break must have happened at the water jump and it was only skin and muscle that had held it together for a few minutes more. It didn't make me feel any better.

I know there are a great deal of animal-rights campaigners that think National Hunt racing is a cruel sport and that all those associated with it have no care for the horses, but nothing, nothing at all, could be further from the truth.

Anyone who has ever ridden will tell you that if a horse doesn't want to jump an obstacle, then there is no way on earth you are going to make it. The ludicrous notion that a jockey, no matter how strong they are, could force a ton or more of horse over a jump is laughable. Watch any National Hunt race to see what happens when the horse decides that they have had enough. If it's at a fence, nine times out of ten they will simply plant their feet and it's the hapless jockey who sails over on his or her own.

Also, while you are watching, look for what happens when a horse loses its jockey. There is no external reason and no requirement for any riderless horse to keep on, yet the majority of them will happily keep running and jumping of their own volition. There are lots of places for them to duck out of the course, so when they decide to go ahead it's because they are enjoying themselves. Add to that the reality that horse racing is the only reason thoroughbred racehorses are bred. If there was no racing, there would be none of these horses in existence. None. Sadly there are some deaths in horse racing, but far more horses, by a massive margin, are killed on the roads each year and indeed, in paddocks. Finally, the idea that those involved in racing somehow don't care is abhorrent. The horses are treated like stars, their accommodation, feed and care is second-to-none and the stable lads and lasses treat them like revered members of their own family. Should tragedy strike, well I have seen grown men and women bawling like babies when one of their horses is injured or killed. I know that even goes for the majority of the race going public. We build such an affinity with our horses that when one is hurt it is like losing a friend. I recall, many years after Kybo's loss, in 2005, watching the racing at Exeter when Best Mate, three times Cheltenham Gold Cup winner, collapsed and died of a suspected heart attack after being pulled up by jockey Paul Carberry. His trainer, Henrietta Knight, my friend Terry Biddlecombe's wife, was heartbroken, as was owner, Jim Lewis.

If anything, all the animal rights campaigners have done in demanding that fences are made smaller, especially at Aintree, is increase the danger because now the horses tend to go faster and it's the speed that kills.

I do wonder why people, with no sense of what they are talking about, shout the loudest.

That day, when Kybo was lost, Josh left the racecourse immediately. I gathered my things together and as I was leaving I heard a second piece of news that almost floored me. Doctor Alun Thomas, the man who had patched up so many of us, the man without whose intervention and swift action I wouldn't be here, a man I called a friend, had died the previous day.

His obituaries in the British Medical Journal and the British Journal of Sport's Medicine couldn't encapsulate the man of course, but went some way to acknowledge him.

"Alun Thomas died in his sleep on January 16ᵗʰ, 1981. He was associated with W. E. Tucker for twelve years at the Clinic in Park Street, London and took over on Bill's retirement. A Barts man, his early interest and training lay in orthopaedics and he had a wide background of experience in the disorders of the musculo-skeletal system. He gave generously of his time and expertise to all connected with sport and was a familiar figure at major events, particularly at Lord's.

He was especially concerned with the equestrian world and many of the leading show jumpers, event riders and jockeys were looked after by Alun. He was a steward of the British Boxing Board of Control and surgeon to the Injured Jockeys Compensation Fund, Wimbledon F.C., Middlesex County Cricket Club and Lord's Cricket Ground.

Alun was a warm hearted man, a splendid companion and an excellent doctor. His unique position in Sports Medicine was reflected in the large attendance at his memorial service and was a fitting tribute to a much loved man and admired friend."

Fittingly, in the week Alun was laid to rest, I had to return to the Royal Marsden to see how far I had come in the battle against the cancer that his swift action had saved me from. This time they put me through a comprehensive set of tests including bloods and an array of lung capacity and capability examinations. I can remember they put me on a treadmill and speeded it up bit by bit. They'd given me a bell to ring when I was too tired to continue. I ended up ringing it eventually because I was bored, so I figured I'd done okay. It was confirmed when I received a written report a few days later. Of all the press cuttings, mementos and memories that I have kept over the years, this letter has become something of a talisman for me.

"Dear Bob,

When we last tested you, a year ago, your lung function was moderately impaired because of the bleomycin. This time there has been a substantial and pleasing improvement such that your lung volumes are normal again and gas transfer is around the lower limits of normal. Moreover, at exercise you were able to do more than almost anyone we've ever tested and even at this high level of exercise the lungs were able to keep the blood fully saturated with oxygen, which is a strong pointer to normal lung function. We can say you have very little residual lung damage from the bleomycin which is pleasing to us too.

One of the assistants told us you gave him three tips but he could not get to the street to go to the betting shop because he was too busy. Imagine how he felt when he heard that two had won and the other horse was second."

The following Monday I had another winner at Fontwell and went, at the insistence of the other fifteen jockeys at the meeting, up to the Anglo American Sporting Club in the Hilton Hotel, Park Lane for what was apparently a boxing dinner in honour of jockeys. In I wandered to discover the whole thing had been set up with me as the single guest of honour. There were about a thousand people in attendance, all in dinner jackets. Derek was there with Howard and all the rest of the Thompson clan. He made a speech and led everyone in a toast and Lord Oaksey presented me with a decanter and glasses. In return I managed to mumble a few words of thanks and an, 'I didn't know this was for me until I saw the menu with my name on the front of it'. It wasn't my best speech, but they generously gave me a rousing round of applause.

A few days later, I headed to Ascot to be reunited with another survivor of his own battles. Aldaniti was back after breaking down at Sandown fifteen months earlier.

φ

Image Set B:

1. The 1981 National – Becher's 1st time, a complete melee as usual.
2. The 1981 National – Becher's 1st time. Believe it or not, No. 23 Cheers, ridden by the great Peter Scudamore didn't fall despite the precarious angle of the landing and went on to be the last of the 12 finishers.
3. 1981 National, Becher's 2nd time. The classic way to land that legend of a fence.
4. 1981 National, Becher's 2nd time. I can perhaps see why some thought Aldaniti was about to come a cropper, but of course he didn't.
5. 1981 National, Becher's 2nd time and it's poor Steve Jobar on Pacify that fell to our right hand side.
6. 1981 National. Just cleared the 3rd last. Two to go. Concentrate Bob! With Royal Mail in pursuit.
7. Newmarket Yard, 1998
8. Painting up my first stables in 1982
9. Tilly, Ali and Henri
10. Jumping for each of the Japanese papers
11. A charity polo match with John Francome and Charles Betz
12. Looking fit in Saratoga
13. With John Hurt and Aldaniti on the set of Champions.
14. Sharing a smile with John Hurt and Lord Lou Grade
15. Her Majesty the Queen, myself, Janette and Simon Massen
16. Me and the great Jonjo O'Neill in a charity legends race

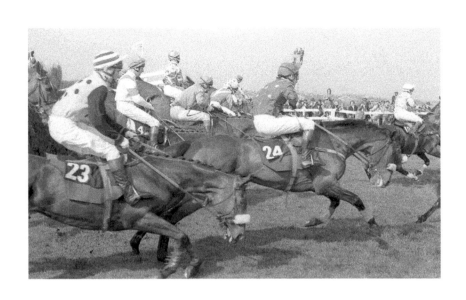

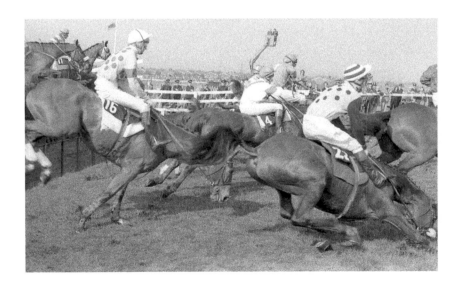

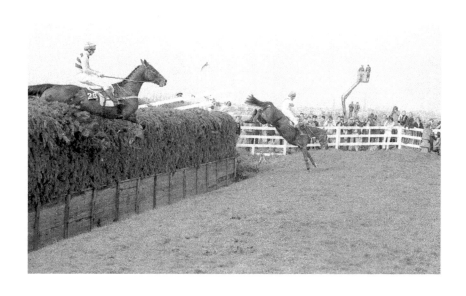

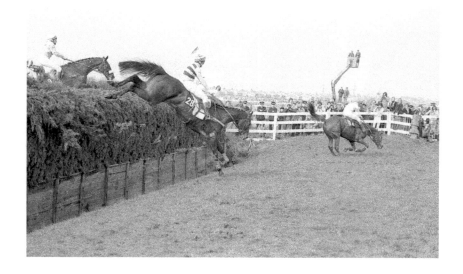

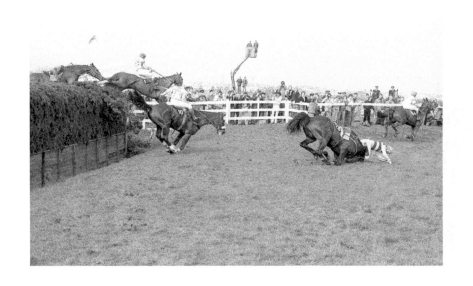

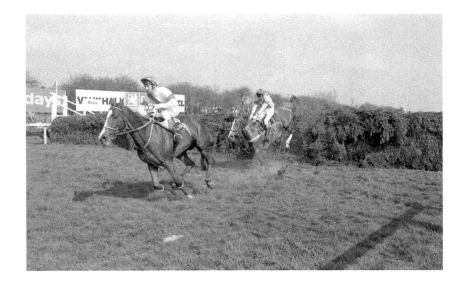

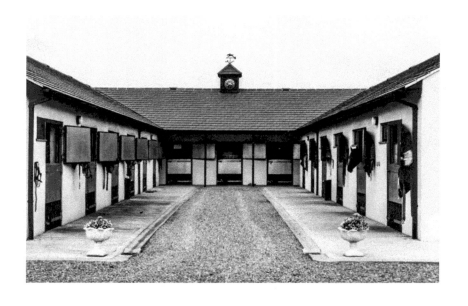

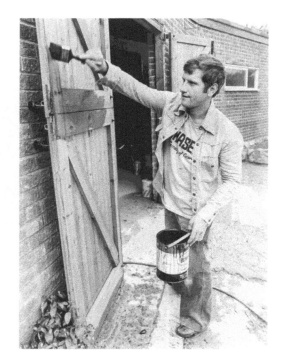

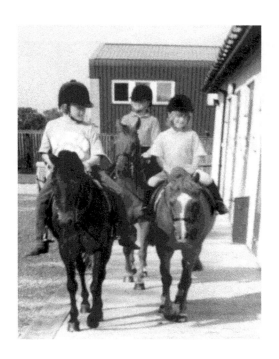

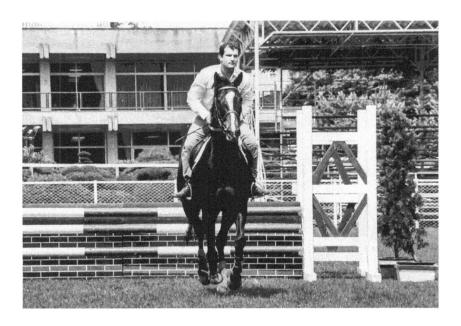

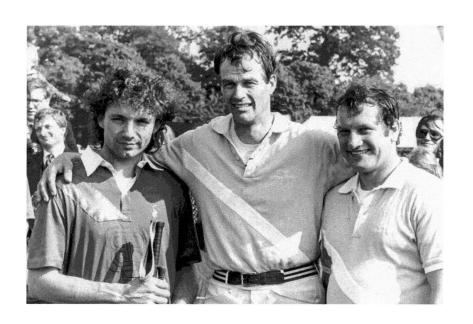

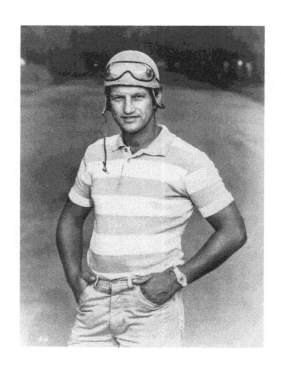

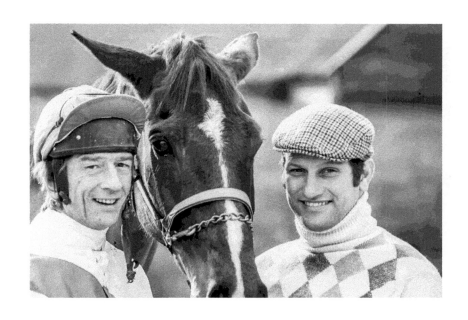

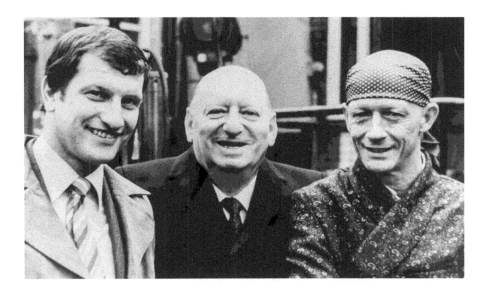

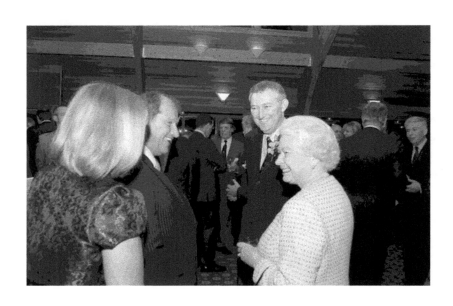

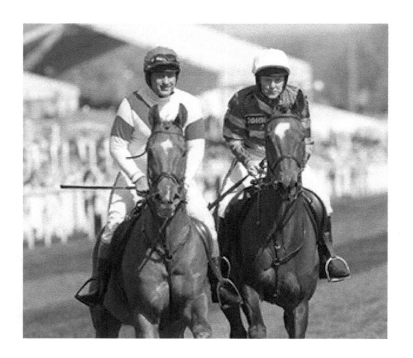

Josh and Nick met me in the paddock but instructions weren't necessary. We all knew Aldaniti had talent but we also knew he'd had some horrendously serious injuries that could well have seen him put down a number of times. All I had to do was take him round nice and gently in the hope that after this, we could prepare him for a shot at the National in April. Most of the bookies must have thought the same as we had started the morning at 33-1. By post time we had shortened to 14s but that was still the longest price in the field of eight that set off in the Whitbread Trial Handicap Chase.

As per usual he jumped superbly well and we settled down at the back. By the time we got to the final mile there were only five left standing and out of them only Cabar Feidh and Royal Charley had any chance of winning. Oh and one other. Aldaniti was travelling as well as I'd ever felt him. I delayed and delayed and let him gain ground over the fences, which he did with every leap. Eventually, at the second last I pressed him to go for the win. I've rarely felt a horse pick up like he did. His reaction was immediate and we stormed home four lengths to the good.

You know when you've ridden a good race, but it's always nice for someone else to tell you. More so when that someone is somebody like Josh Gifford, who you'll recall was himself a four times Champion Jockey. So for him to say that it was the best ride he'd ever seen anyone give a horse was quite a compliment. He went on to say that he would check out Aldaniti's legs over the following seventy-two hours, but if he'd come through all right then there would be no need to run him again. The next time we'd see him would be at Aintree for the National. I personally couldn't wait. But before I would reunite with him, I had a run of success that was unprecedented in my career, accompanied by the most significant test of my post-chemo recovery.

φ

February 1981 was wintery in the extreme and heavy snows cancelled a number of meetings. Despite the limited opportunities, I notched up thirteen winners and in one particular week scored seven from nine rides, amassing a total prize fund of almost £2,000, a colossal weekly income at the time. It seemed like every horse I got on either won, or was placed. I was on a roll, yet all the way through the month I was also more and more aware of the massive test that was coming up at the Royal Marsden. There were no MRIs back then, well, none in mainstream hospitals, so this was to be a full body X-ray examination, by far the most detailed since I'd had the chemo. It was designed to examine in extra detail every inch of me to make sure there were no more cancer cells present. Like every other time, the closer the tests got, the more I worried. This time, my now long-term girlfriend, Jo, bore the brunt of my anxiety.

I stayed overnight with Derek in London and in the morning, headed to the hospital on my own. I could write in here that I was worried and quiet and not looking forward to it. The truth is, I was scared. Simple as that.

The X-ray machine was a long tube, not unlike an MRI, but it was enclosed and only my head popped out the top. Every twenty seconds I had to hold my breath as another image was taken. The whole thing lasted two hours. When it was complete, I went up to the ward to say hello to the patients and nurses, then drove home. The following day I was back. Once more it was Doctor Jane that gave me the news. Once more, it was fantastic. Once more, she confirmed I was completely cancer-free. Not only that, but I wouldn't need to come back for any more tests for three months. I was so happy and when I got home, the news just kept getting better. For the second time in three months I'd been chosen as the Amoco Jockey of the Month. It was unprecedented for a jockey to have won it twice in such a timescale and I was really pleased. The Sporting Life ran an article under the headline, 'Five Star Champion'. I'd have thought four star for the petrol connection would have been better, but at least they had given up on the whole Champion the Wonder Horse analogy. In the March I rode Approaching in the Cheltenham Gold Cup but made no impression in the race. I wasn't bothered. All of my attention was now on Aintree, although in the immediate run up to it the chance to ride Aldaniti was almost snatched away, had it not been for a friendly police officer.

With four days to go before the start of the National meeting, Josh had received a call from the local police telling him that there had been an outbreak of Foot and Mouth in the local area and they were going to have to seal off the village of Findon. As soon as they put the quarantine into place, nothing could move in or out. They knew what Josh's plans were and so they advised that if Aldaniti was going to go to Aintree, best he go now. Thankfully, due to their timely warning we were able to move him up to Liverpool early. Thinking we'd dodged a bullet, we gathered on the Thursday for the first race of the meeting. It was to be the worst possible start.

Nick and Valda owned a string of horses and one of them, Stonepark, was entered to run in the Topham Trophy with Richard Rowe on board. The Topham is run over the National fences and is a good test of a horse. Stonepark was a consistent type and went off as one of the favourites. Despite this, he fell at the first and although he struggled back up to his feet, it was obvious that he was seriously injured. Richard couldn't catch him and Stonepark set off riderless. When he was eventually caught the course vet determined that he had broken his neck in the fall. There was nothing to be done for him and Stonepark was subsequently put down.

The loss was a huge blow for Valda. She was overcome with grief and Nick decided that he couldn't risk losing Aldaniti in a similar way. He decided to pull him from the National. It was a perfectly understandable reaction, but after a short while Nick decided that he owed it to everyone involved to go ahead.

The day had been a bad one already, but personally mine was about to get worse. It almost got an awful lot worse. I had a ride on Kilbrony in the last race of the day and at the water jump he stood off too far, ended up dropping into the water, slipped, rolled and put me face first into the turf. Nothing too unusual, I lay still and waited for the other runners to pass me by, but I ended up being run over and trampled like a ball in a child's rugby scrum. One of the back markers, Sunrise Hill, kicked out on his way past. I felt the closeness of one of his hooves as it missed my head by inches, the other hit me square in the back and for one moment I thought I'd had it. I really thought he'd broken me in two. After a while I managed to pull myself up and limp back to the changing room. When

I stripped my colours off there was a great big red hoof print in the middle of my back. In a way, I was a little relieved. What with my fantastic run of form, I hadn't had a fall in weeks. I thought perhaps it was a good thing to get one in early. I knew that a couple of paracetamol, a sauna, a plunge pool and a massage would see me right as rain. I told the course doctor I was fine and he agreed. I had one ride on the Friday, finishing unplaced in a novice hurdle and was happy that my back, although a bit stiff, had come through it okay. That night I appeared on TV a couple of times in pre-recorded interviews and in a 'Grand National Special' edition of the popular quiz show, A Question of Sport, then I headed to bed.

I had made it back. I was on the eve of riding Aldaniti in the Grand National. This was what had seen me through the whole of my ordeal. This was what I had told everyone I was going to do. Now it was time to prove to everyone that I'd been right.

The 1981
Grand National

To describe the Grand National as a horse race is like describing a Rolls Royce as a car or Concorde as an aeroplane. Better still, it's like saying the Ashes is just a cricket match or the FA Cup Final, just a kick-about. Factually all correct, but just not getting the idea at all.

The National is a British icon and by far the most prominent horse race in British culture, potentially in international racing culture. Each year, on that one day, millions of people who wouldn't normally bet or show an interest in horse racing, have a flutter and watch the television coverage.

Statistically, it is the richest jump race held in Europe with a prize fund that is now in excess of £1M. Properly described as a handicap steeplechase, run over 4miles 514yards around Aintree, it's usually held on the first weekend in April. Inaugurated in 1839, the course is not only long, but the 30 fences jumped during the two circuits are much bigger obstacles than those found on conventional National Hunt courses. Many of them are famous in their own right, such as the Canal Turn, Valentine's, The Chair and the most famous of all, Becher's Brook. All in all, this single horse race has, through the size of the fences, the distance run and the enormity of its history, earned its title of 'the ultimate test of horse and rider.'

For me it was a lot less complicated.

It was my greatest ambition in life, since I was eight, to ride in a National. One of my biggest thrills was the first time I ever got round, on Hurricane Rock. But to win one? Well… that was the stuff of dreams. A dream that I was part of.

Aintree, Liverpool, the 4th April 1981. Under the canopy of an azure sky, thirty-nine horses, their shadows sharply defined by a bright spring sun, lined up for the biggest test in British racing.

Me, recovered and racing fit. Aldaniti, after breaking down at Sandown in November 1979, recovered and racing fit. It was a seemingly impossible story. But here we were.

For my part, I felt magnificent and was amazed by Aldaniti. I'd never known him to handle the way he did when I rode him out that morning. He was calm, assured. I know it sounds like I'm making it up in hindsight, but I was so confident. In fact, I was sure; we were going to win this.

I got my final instructions from Josh as he gave me the leg-up into the saddle.

"Hold him up Bob, give him a breather, sit and don't hit the front until going to the last fence."

I think I nodded and agreed, "No problem Guv'nor. I have this. We're going to win this. You should have no worries."

Josh looked up to me, "Why are you so sure?"

"He'll win it, I'm telling you!"

I can now admit what I didn't tell Josh or anyone else back then; the previous time I'd ridden Aldaniti, I'd been several pounds heavier than the weight I should have been and he'd still won. This time I was spot on my declared weight.

Before Josh leant down to do a final check of the girths he had to get rid of the almost constant cigarette in his hand. The man smoked like the proverbial train and I said, "Hey Guv'nor, if I win today will you give up smoking?"

He looked up at me and with almost no hesitation said, "Yes. You win and I'll give them up." He was always a man of his word and sure enough he did as he promised.

Then it was down to me to settle myself. Deal with the long build up. The long parade. Canter down to the first fence, let Aldaniti have a look at it, a sniff of the spruce. Let him pop his head up and over it. Then back to the start. Circling and waiting. I manoeuvred around and picked my place on the outside of the field. Josh and I had figured the outside was firmer ground. I could see others, including John Francome, opting for a different line. Tucking into what would be the inside rail meant less congestion, but also the fences dropped away more in there. It was, quite literally a case of horses for courses.

I concentrated on my position, watching the rest of the runners around me. Even in a big field you know the horses. You've studied the form book and it never lies. You know the jockeys. You work with them every day. Looking up, watching the starter, each one of them with their own foibles. Each one different. Turning again, round in a wide arc, watching, keeping your position, feeling the anticipation of the crowd building, feeling the buzz spreading throughout the jockeys, trying to keep your own emotions settled. Not passing them to the horse. Watching, waiting. Making sure we kept within the starter's guidance. Listening to his commands to turn and step up. Thinking about Josh's instructions. 'Hold him, Bob. Hold him.' I have this.

But after Captain Dick Smalley raised the tapes and sent us on our way, things didn't quite go to plan.

The start was accompanied by the cheers of a 50,000 strong crowd, the thundering of 156 hooves and the raw power of almost eighteen tons of horse flesh pounding down to the first fence. I'd been here before, eight times before. I was one of the 'old hands' now. The sure and certain knowledge that most runners hit the first travelling far too fast was uppermost in my mind, so I wanted to hold back. Not be in the front-most wave. I tried to walk Aldaniti through the tapes, but he was off and running at once.

It's a quarter of a mile to the first fence which sounds far, but takes no time at all at racing pace. Halfway there you cross the cinder track of the Melling Road. I'd been told by Fred Winter, winner of two Nationals, to take a pull as soon as I crossed it, which I did, though I figured we were still going at a fair gallop. Despite trying to rein him in, Aldaniti came to the first travelling far too quickly. He stood way off, cleared it but landed steeply. I slipped my reins to the buckle and seriously thought, 'Bugger, we're gone, what a bloody waste.'

He was down, almost flat on his belly on the ground, and still now I'm not sure how he managed to recover, but he did. I regained my balance and thought that perhaps the experience might calm him down a little, but he went into the second equally fast, stood off it even more than the first and came so close to landing on top of it that he scraped his belly. It hurt him and I thought that might have taught him a lesson. I never felt like falling that time, but I reckoned, if the horse didn't get a grip of this, then it wouldn't be that long before the inevitable happened.

The third fence is that massive ditch and I felt Aldaniti's surprise. It might even have been a little bit of fear, but he was nothing if not brave and he went into it without so much as a flinch.

We got to the fourth and I remember having to squeeze him a little but that was when the penny dropped. He had sorted himself out. Obviously he'd thought about the first three obstacles and from the fourth onwards, he was sound. In fact, he was superb. From then on all I had to do was ride him at the fence and he'd come up for me. He was a joy. I just had to stay with him. You see the horse was not only brave, he was intelligent. He'd been having a look at the fences and, as he'd never fallen in his life, he quickly figured out that he needed to be closer in to them. He needed to pop over them rather than stretch for them.

We settled into a good rhythm but as per usual there were fallers all around us. Two had gone at the first, then two refused and one fell at the fourth. The fifth was cleared by all and then it was up to Becher's Brook. Nowadays Becher's has been modified extensively, yet it is still a formidable obstacle. When I ran the race it was even more daunting. The fence itself, at 4ft 10in doesn't seem all that big in comparison, but the landing side falls away and back in 1981, that fall away was in the order of a three foot drop. It's like jumping off the edge of the world. Most horses are not expecting it and the rider has to sit well back and use their weight as ballast. Combine all of that with a left hand turn immediately after it and you can see why it was considered the most thrilling and famous fence in the horse racing world. It was also responsible for a lot of fallers in most years.

Amazingly, all bar one cleared it this time. We went over back in about 29th place, then the whole field cleared the seventh. At the Canal Turn (8) our racing line was good and by Valentine's (9) we had jumped to contest the lead about three and a half miles earlier than planned. I just had to adapt. To be honest, I was basically controlling the pace of the race for the rest of it so I wasn't that worried. I had faith in Aldaniti.

In fact, after we had come second in the 1979 Scottish Grand National, I'd wondered if I should have allowed him to take up the running earlier that day. So there we were, halfway round the first circuit, cleared Becher's, made a lot of ground up over the Canal Turn and after the leader, Carrow Boy, fell at the tenth, Aldaniti and I were basically second. Another open ditch and we were neck and neck for the lead with Sebastian V (a former fourth placed in the National), a good proven jumper and steady runner. I tried to hold Aldaniti, but he was still surging. Yet even then, I was still comfortable with how we were going. I know some horses wouldn't have been keen, that far in front with another circuit and more to go, but Aldaniti had spent so long recovering from his injuries, I knew he had the patience to sit there and wait. I also knew from riding him that morning that he was so relaxed. I remember thinking that horses will either adapt to Liverpool or they won't and Aldaniti, out in front so early, was adapting wonderfully.

But I also knew Josh wouldn't have been feeling so pleased with my position. If I did go on to lose, he'd have given me a right bollocking for being at the front so early. The truth was I had gotten there without really trying. Aldaniti was so keen to get on with it and I just had to cope with him now.

It's a strange thing that happened at that point and I know some may wonder at it, but I began to recollect former Nationals. I remembered Red Rum and how he had won, I thought about the horses around me and whether they'd had good or bad runs previously. I was able to consider the likely opposition in the closing stages. Simply put, I had a lot of time to think and it was because the riding part of my brain was off doing its own thing. I know it sounds a little strange, but I reckon it would be summed up nowadays as me being in 'the Zone'. Aldaniti and I were operating on a different level and by the next fence we were in the lead. No longer did I have the option of settling him behind another runner, so I hoped he would settle by himself out front. He didn't. He nearly pulled the arms out of me with his head swinging from side to side, though the one thing I wasn't worried about was my strength failing. I was as strong as I'd ever been. All that training in America had been worth it.

A few more fences, a few more fallers and then it was the Chair (15). The biggest obstacle on the course, and lots of people have asked me, "What do you think about, travelling at the speed you are and approaching a monster of a fence like that?" The truth is, you don't think about it. You just ride the horse and with Aldaniti that day he took the inside line, saw a nice long stride, stood off it and really pinged over it. There are photos I've seen and I'm sitting up his neck like a flat jockey. He cleared it easily, making ground up with the jump. Now, as well as Sebastian V, Rubstic, a former winner, was on our outer, with Zongalero and Royal Stuart pegging us back.

Royal Stuart took a marginal lead for a while after the Water (16) but as we headed out into the country for the second circuit, I could feel Aldaniti's strength. He was loving the run and I knew, if I could keep him safe, he'd see me home. I knew it. What I didn't know was dear old John Thorne on the favourite, Spartan Missile, was not going to let it be that easy.

We crossed the Melling Road and went to the 17th where we had the lead from Rubstic by half a length, but Aldaniti put in a majestic jump and we landed three lengths in front. The next four fences were cleared with what seemed no effort at all. He popped them and there was literally nothing else near us. We had daylight all around.

Coming into Becher's for the second time, I swung him out to the middle of the track and then angled him in to take it on the inside and save a bit of distance. I've never jumped it better. Some journalists said later that it looked like Aldaniti had come a cropper and it was my 'excellent horsemanship' that had kept him in the race. I thought that was nonsense. Yes, we pitched as you always do on the drop side, but his head came up straight away and what with the then second placed, Pacify and Steve Jobar falling to my right, we were five or six lengths to the good. Zongalero and Steve Smith-Eccles also went there and in truth there were very few that stood any chance from here on, but those that did were prepared to make a race of it.

I took Aldaniti wide at the Canal Turn, keeping it safe and stood off Valentine's a bit. Five from home and seemingly out of nowhere, but with a brave effort, Royal Mail had almost come alongside us. Going to the fourth last and I know now that John Thorne and Spartan Missile were also beginning to make their way through the remaining runners, but in 1981, all I actually knew was that I had to concentrate on my race. Think like a professional jockey. Do not get caught up in the realisation that I might actually win this. For real. I know I had said I was convinced we would, but this was actually happening.

The third last and it was us, closely pressed by Royal Mail, about six or seven lengths to Three-to-One in third, fourth was Senator Maclacury and Spartan Missile was just passing the mighty Rubstic.

I could feel Aldaniti, he hadn't faltered once. His legs were good. I knew he'd keep galloping, but as we'd gone to that third last I couldn't see a stride, so I'd let him drift. It was when we landed that I was really aware of Royal Mail pressing down on us.

There's such a long run up to the second last and I kept telling myself to stop thinking about winning. Just concentrate and take the proper line. Josh and I had discussed it, keep him wide and seek out the better ground.

We approached the fence with about two lengths on Royal Mail and Phillip Blacker (who had headed us in the Cheltenham Gold Cup) and Aldaniti put in another terrific jump. We opened another length and then I heard a crash immediately behind. Royal Mail had gone straight through it and made a terrible peck on landing. Once more we had clear space around us.

Phillip rallied Royal Mail yet again on the approach to the last, my goodness when you watch the race back, that horse had some stamina and powers of recovery and I wonder if he hadn't made such a bad mistake at the second last could things have been closer, but at the time it was of no concern. We strode into the last and put in another good jump. We were over. No more obstacles. As long as we didn't do a 'Devon Loch' all we had left was the longest run-in in English racing. Another 474yards to glory.

Royal Mail rallied yet again to within two lengths and I could see him on my right. I gave Aldaniti just a couple of reminders and he went again with a speed that surprised even me. We left Royal Mail another two lengths in our wake. I thought that was the end of the opposition, but I wasn't aware that Spartan Missile and the gentleman John Thorne were reeling us in quickly. I hit 'The Elbow' and went into the last furlong three lengths to the good. Aldaniti rolled a bit left, as if he was heading back to the Chair, and I corrected him, but at that point in the run-in there are no running rails to help guide the horse. I could feel now he was desperately tired and that never-ending run-in at Aintree has seen the undoing of many a great horse. I'd seen Red Rum destroy Crisp and I was determined that wasn't going to happen. I wished I could see behind me but I was damned if I was going to look.

Three-quarters of a furlong to go and now I was certainly aware someone was catching me up. I could sense them just over my right shoulder. I thought it was Royal Mail coming again, but it wasn't. Later on I'd learn it had been John on Spartan Missile. They'd made an amazing effort. He'd come off the final fence ten lengths or more behind us and yet was running like he was on his first circuit.

But at the time, it didn't matter who it was. I had half a furlong left and there's far too much noise from the crowd at that point to know exactly what's going on behind you, so all I could do was keep riding, but I could feel the other horse drawing nearer. It was definitely closing with what seemed like every stride and the winning post seemed to be going away instead of getting nearer. I remember going to give Aldaniti another reminder but I didn't need to. He too had sensed the nearing threat and responded with just my hands and heels. He accelerated again. All I had to do was stay in the saddle. I waved the whip in my right hand for encouragement, gave him a couple of slaps with my left hand on his neck and felt the distance growing between me and my pursuer. With five yards to what I always called, 'the lollypop', I finally knew I had it in the bag. As we passed the winning post with four lengths to spare, I raised my hand in salute to the Grandstand and the cheers of the crowd.

We'd just won the Grand National!

It was my boyhood dream fulfilled. It was the goal I had set myself, to survive everything the chemo had thrown at me. It was the day the rest of my life started. At that moment Aldaniti and I were one. Great clouds of steam were rising off him, sweat was pouring off me. My adrenaline rush and his were combined in an exquisite moment of partnership. Two broken beings, written off, unlikely to survive, told time and again we'd never make it back, had come together in that one amazing moment. In the immediate afterglow of my victory I decided to retire from National Hunt. I'd leave at the moment of my greatest triumph. Before I had even dismounted from Aldaniti in the winner's enclosure I had changed my mind. I remember thinking, 'No way am I calling it a day. I want to do this again.' In hindsight, that was a mistake.

Slowing to a canter and then to a walk I sat down in the saddle just as Snowy, the travelling head lad and Pete Double, a stable jockey who was such a talent but never got the opportunities, caught me up and took the reins of Aldaniti. Both of them were laughing and smiling and slapping Aldaniti on the neck. They led me round and I felt a hand on my left shoulder. It was John Thorne. He clapped me on the back and told me, "Well done Bob, you deserve it, great ride, well done." What an absolute gent he was.

Snowy and Pete led me towards the winner's enclosure and by now a number of other people associated with the yard and the horse were gathering round. We were stopped momentarily by the pressing of the crowd wanting to wish us well and that's the moment I will never forget. It's imprinted into me and had the most 'physical' impact on me out of all the swirling memories of that day. I can probably say without being overly dramatic, it was, and is, the most iconic moment of my life.

You see, when I was a young boy dreaming of winning the National and ever since then, when I imagined it, envisioned it and focussed on it through the long, bleak days of my illness, the picture was always the same. It wasn't the tapes going up, nor jumping Becher's, nor galloping up the Elbow and past the winning post. No, it was only ever the one image. The thing, which to me, always captured the aura of the winning jockey and horse in the Aintree Grand National. It was the simple act of mounted police riders coming to flank the victors.

I looked right and left and felt a lump in my throat. We'd done it and I was in the middle of my dream image. Aldaniti, glistening with sweat and the police horses, four calm and serene bays walking alongside, gently nudging a clearway for us to proceed. Once through the tight tangle of people we made our way down the narrow approach to the winner's enclosure. Halfway there Josh and Nick stepped out to join us. Nick took the reins and led Aldaniti, the horse he and his wife Valda had put their faith and trust into, the horse they hadn't destroyed as so many others would have, to the Grand National Winner's spot.

As I dismounted I could see that Josh, who was quite an emotional man, had a tear in his eye. Emotional or not, he very rarely gave out praise, so I was chuffed when he reached out, took my hand and said, "Well done." From the man who had never broken his word about keeping me as his jockey, all through the trials and tribulations of my illness, the praise meant a lot. As did looking up and seeing Mr McKenzie, my old school teacher, who had always known I would be a jockey. From the side of the enclosure he gave me a smile and a nod of his head. I returned his smile, but was almost brought to tears when I caught the eye of both Jenny and Carol from the Royal Marsden. They'd sacrificed one of their holiday days just to be there for me and that they could share in my triumph meant so much to me. I felt a lump in my throat and a welling up of immense gratitude.

Then I had David Coleman from the BBC right in front of me with a microphone and as he spoke to me we watched the tail end of the race on a small TV monitor. That's when I found out it had been John and Spartan Missile pursuing us. I was so chuffed at how we'd won. Aldaniti had been magnificent. Coleman asked me to sum up my thoughts and perhaps it was seeing Jenny and Carol or perhaps it was just a bit of divine inspiration, but I'm quite proud of what I came up with. It's still as true now as it was then when I said, "I rode this race for all the patients in hospital and all the people that look after them. My only wish is that my winning shows them that there is always hope, and all battles can be won. I just hope I will encourage others to face their illness with fresh spirit."

I finally made the weighing room and thankfully weighed in the same as I'd weighed out. The valet, 'Pipe-smoking Robin', who had travelled up especially for me, took my saddle and started the job of getting everything ready for the next race. Usually I'd have followed him into the changing room, but this time my way was cut off by what looked like hundreds of cameras and a mass of press reporters, TV reporters and radio broadcasters from what seemed like every nation on earth. In fact my only regret that day, was that I never got back into the changing room at that time to feel the atmosphere in there. It was always fantastic after the National. The camaraderie and banter were to the fore, and the champagne was always flowing, but I missed it because I was caught up in a blizzard of interviews. Various people did try to offer me a celebratory glass, but every time I was given champagne, a photographer took it out of my hand. I think the first drink I got was a can of coke, hours later heading back down the motorway. I was gasping.

Eventually though, I managed to detach myself from the press in just enough time to get changed for the last race on the card that day. National Hunt jockeys rarely get to rest on any laurels, even the biggest ones, so an hour and a half later, after the greatest triumph of my life, I was back at the starting line in a novice hurdle. On a horse called Homeson, I finished a fairly okay fifth. Josh met me back in the unsaddling enclosure and gave me a right bollocking about the way I had ridden. I think it was just to keep me grounded and stop me thinking I was God's gift. National Hunt racing is quite the leveller.

φ

On the way home I stopped at a service station on the M6 to call Mary. It was the first chance I had and I wanted to hear what my family thought. It was such a good feeling to know that everyone was so incredibly proud. Poor Mum had been unable to watch the whole of the race and had hidden behind the kitchen door, peering round until she could stand it no longer and had to look away completely. Mary said that watching it at home was far better as they got to see the whole of the race and could tell me far more about it. I knew they'd all had bets on me so I was certainly in their good books!

A group of us stopped with John Thorne in a restaurant in Stratford. We had a great evening and got home at midnight. I was up again by six, so as to get down to Findon to see Aldaniti returning home. It's a tradition, like the winning team of the FA Cup final parading the trophy. The morning after the big race, people come from all over the country just to welcome back the National winner. Findon isn't that big a village, so it was a bit surprising to see thousands of people gathered along the streets. I mean you'd seen big turnouts when Red Rum had returned home, but this seemed to be even bigger than that. It was my first inclination that Aldaniti and I might have struck a chord with the public because of our story. Josh and Nick decided to let Aldaniti out about half a mile from the yard, Pete led him and we walked alongside so that everyone who had made the effort could see him.

As I walked Aldaniti toward the stables, with his ears pricked and his head looking from side to side, I recalled a conversation that Josh and I had had the evening before in the Stratford restaurant. Josh had said that Aldaniti and I had joined together to put up a staggering performance. He said that I had given Aldaniti the most brilliant ride. It was nice of him to say it and I certainly appreciated his praise, but to me it was easier than that. Aldaniti was unbelievably tough. I always knew he would keep going until he dropped and honestly, even now after all these years, I know had you planted a twenty-foot brick wall in front of him that day, he'd have gone straight through it. He was exhausted at the end, but however tired he'd have kept galloping for another ten miles. It was his guts that won the race, nothing else.

φ

Had you asked what I expected to happen following my win I'd have said I honestly had no clue. I'd been so focused on the race itself, I hadn't considered the aftermath. I'll also admit, that even when I was imagining and envisioning my win, even while desperately wanting it, I don't think I fully accepted I would. Well, you don't. It's sort of like the lottery. You keep hoping and praying you'll win, you might even picture it in your mind's eye, but you don't think it will happen. Turned out that basically, I was quite good at hoping, but I hadn't thought past that hope.

As it was, the immediate aftermath of winning the National was, for me, what I imagine an athlete would feel like after winning a gold at the Olympic Games, or a boxer, the World Heavyweight Championship. It was the ultimate pinnacle of my chosen sport. The race that I'd always wanted to win. I was so, so lucky to have done it, especially when you consider the really great, legendary jockeys who never had any luck at Liverpool. I didn't really, deep down believe it was true until we passed the post and even now, sometimes, I still have to remind myself it was real.

With my focus having been on the race for so long, once it ended I suppose I could have expected a hiatus of everything really. It turned out, there was no time for a break. That morning arriving at Findon had given me an inkling, but I was surprised at the scale of the fuss that was caused. Don't get me wrong, I'm not being overly coy, I understood that Aldaniti and I had overcome huge adversity, but for me I was simply doing the job that I loved on a horse I adored. I didn't feel like I'd done the hard work. For me, Josh and Nick and all the team had done the real graft in getting Aldaniti ready for the race. It wasn't about my courage, it was about riding the best race of my life.

So when the term National Hero started being thrown about, I wasn't comfortable at all. The only way I ended up accepting it was when it was put in the context of being an inspiration to those patients who felt they had no hope. I was more than happy for the whole experience to be presented as that. If I could help anyone who was going through what I had, then I was all for it. I still didn't realise how much my story had impacted the public in general.

The first week after the race was a bit of a blur and as a shy man at heart, the invasive interest of the press was hard to take. There were some times that I wondered at the questions I was being asked and often thought people must be bored with seeing my face plastered all over the TV and newspapers. Thankfully we didn't have the internet then or I'd never have escaped seeing myself. I'd have gone viral!

It took maybe two weeks until the full enormity of what Aldaniti and I had done began to be revealed. By that time, the mail had begun to arrive in earnest. I received some incredible letters and telegrams, the majority of which I still have today. I was so humbled and I am more than happy and proud to admit that I framed the letters from the Queen Mother and Prince Charles.

The Queen Mother's personal secretary Sir Martin Gilliat wrote, *"I am delighted to convey to you Queen Elizabeth, The Queen Mother's warmest congratulations on your wonderful victory. Your success brought to Her Majesty enormous pleasure as it undoubtedly did to millions in all parts of the world."*

Whilst Prince Charles wrote, whilst on his hectic visits to New Zealand and Australia, *"I simply had to write a short letter of admiration following your wonderful win in the Grand National. It really was the best possible news after your illness and the troubles with Aldaniti. I am so glad that fate has been so generous to you at last. With my very best wishes and renewed congratulations. Charles."*

This letter was particularly special knowing that Charles himself had ridden steeplechase in the previous months. He knew firsthand how much courage and determination was required, to not only race but to win.

I read the letter from Doctor Jane with a particular warmth, as, if not for her persuasion, I would not have been here to race at all. *"Congratulations on winning the race and the fight. We are all delighted."*

For me though, I began to properly realise that this was about giving hope to others and the letter I think that touched me the most at the time, was from a lady in Norfolk. *"Thank you for winning the Grand National. Thank you from someone who spends much of her time nursing cancer patients. Your achievement on Saturday will give cancer sufferers all over the world terrific encouragement and a great deal of hope. Your courage and fortitude will be a terrific boost for people at this present time undergoing depressive chemotherapy and cancer operations."*

It was also then that we learnt people had spontaneously been sending money to the Royal Marsden, care of Bob Champion. Some had sent their winnings from the race, some had sent a separate donation. Some sent pennies, some sent pounds. The doctors called me up and said, "Bob, we should have a talk about what to do."

Around this whirlwind of a time I also decided to marry my then girlfriend Jo. This might seem like a strange thing to do when so much was going on, but I loved her and wanted to spend my life with her, so what better time to do it.

I can look back now and see the National victory as a watershed in my life. Until April 1981 I really had only one focus. Plenty of distractions, but one focus; I was a jump jockey who rode horses. From the moment I passed the winning post at Aintree, I was going to be pulled in three different directions. At times, especially during the first half of the 1980s, I felt like the only jockey in a 3-horse race. Even now, trying to separate and make sense out of what came next is difficult, and I was there! To try to explain it to you as a single whole story would be confusing, so I've decided to give each distinct part its own chapter. I hope it'll make better sense this way.

A Show
Pony

The first and most dramatic change came with the wave of publicity that followed the race. It seemed that I had become 'Public Property' and every news outlet and media channel wanted a piece of me. That wave wasn't going to lessen for some considerable time and all of a sudden I realised it was time for me to grow up. I was going to be much more visible than ever before and somehow that came with extra responsibilities.

I found myself in a world to which I was not familiar, nor comfortable and I had to learn fast. I needed to gain a new outward confidence that would be a front for my shyness. Something robust enough that I could hide behind. It wasn't an easy time but to be honest I was swept along and just had to go with it. One of the main things that was to consume my time and one that at first I had laughed about, was the idea of a book about my life. It was a strange notion that anyone would want to read about me, but even before the National, there had been a lot of talk about me writing a book. Several people had asked and I was getting letters from publishers asking me to consider their proposals. I kept throwing them away.

However, by 1980 the first solid idea of a biography came about. To be honest I was taken aback and actually said to my friend Jonathan Powell, a racing correspondent, that it was a stupid idea.

"I mean, who on earth wants to read about a jockey who's had cancer and wants to make it back into racing?"

He thought quietly for several minutes and then said, "You know what, Bob? That's not such a silly idea."

I told him if he wanted to write it I'd help him as best I could. At least I knew Jonathan, we went to races together and so I knew we would get on okay. I was away working on my fitness in the US but gave him as much help as possible.

The original concept was that Jonathan would write my story from my earliest days through to my comeback into racing after the cancer treatment. As time went on he decided that the final chapter would be the 1981 National, regardless of the outcome. He even arranged for the photographer, Jack Knight, to be at the finishing line to take my picture as I crossed. It was a bold plan and because he had all the rest of it completed, the book was going to be ready to come out very shortly after the race. Of course, none of us could have figured that we would get a fairy-tale ending. That was just the proverbial icing on the cake. To be honest, I never thought a book could come about so quickly, but Jonathan was dogged in his determination and worked extremely hard on it. Due to his efforts the book, *Champion's Story–A Great Human Triumph by Bob Champion and Jonathan Powell, printed by Fontana Paperbacks* was released in the autumn of 1981 at a special launch in Covent Garden at which Aldaniti was in attendance. However, even before it had come out, I'd been completely blown away by another couple of approaches.

On the Sunday immediately after the National, I got a call from Disney Studios about a film. Now this really was laughable. A book was one thing but a movie? Don't be daft!

Yet it seemed that the win had changed everything. A number of media companies knew a book was in the works, now it appeared that a movie was a done deal. Although Disney called first, I was so glad it wasn't them that eventually made it as I don't think I'd have looked good as a cartoon. Besides, Americans can't make racing movies and we didn't need another National Velvet! So a few more weeks passed and then I was told that Lord Lew Grade was going to make it happen. Apparently he was looking for something to get his teeth into after the relative failure of Raise the Titanic in 1980, a film he had famously commented on by saying, "It would have been cheaper to lower the Atlantic." Keen to get a quick success, he got Ladbrokes Entertainment Ltd to sponsor 'Champions' and when they agreed, off we went. Next thing I knew John Hurt had been signed up. That was quite amazing. Can you imagine, John Hurt playing me? These things just don't happen to a Yorkshire jockey! John was a truly fantastic actor and in the three years prior to my National win he'd been in Midnight Express and the Elephant Man, for which he'd been nominated for an Oscar on each occasion. He'd also been in that most memorable scene from Alien, when the little baby alien breaks out of Kane's chest. All of that and now he was going to be me. I wondered if the film's producers had lost their marbles.

As the months wore on I learned more and more about the casting and about the whole of the movie process. We had the lovely Jan Francis playing my wife, Jo and Edward Woodward was going to be Josh Gifford. I'm not sure if Josh was more impressed than me at that news.

Meeting Kirstie Alley, who played the US vet that advised me to get checked out, was a pleasure too. She was even lovelier in person than you see on the screen and I wish I'd been as lucky to date someone that beautiful in reality! Kirstie was the proof to me that true stars were generous with their time and completely down-to-earth and charming. You couldn't have got further from the idea of a Hollywood 'diva'.

If I'm completely honest I was more than a little enamoured by Jan Francis. She was absolutely gorgeous looking and as sweet as the sitcom 'Girl-next-door' characters that she portrayed. She was going to be playing my soon to be wife, Jo, but in real life she was already happily married herself, so that was as far as my infatuation got! The fantastic and hilarious Alison Steadman played my sister Mary and I think she did a fantastic job of showing Mary's bossy nature. Not that I said that to Mary at the time.

I can, hand on heart, say that all of the actors and actresses were really good. I don't think it can be easy playing someone who's not only a real person, but in our case, someone who was still alive. They had to balance the need to get the vital characteristics, but without being a mimic or an impressionist. It was fascinating to see how they would talk things over with John Irvine, the director and then they would take another go at the scene, incorporating whatever changes they had decided. It was very dynamic and quite a fluid process. I was impressed.

Looking back, 1983, or 'My Movie Year' as I came to think about it, was, to coin a cliché, a rollercoaster. I went through so many highs and lows but overall, it was an amazing experience that I wouldn't have missed for anything.

I spent a lot of time initially with the script writer, Evan Jones, to make sure the story as it had been adapted from the book was accurate. Obviously a movie script needs to be cut down substantially from a book and as writers do, for dramatic purposes, he wanted to embellish bits. I feared he and the rest of the movie 'execs' would be very demanding and inflexible, yet they were actually very comfortable when I pushed back. For example, to add a bit of tension and gravitas into an early part of the film, they wanted to portray me as a boozer. Now, I'm a lot of things, but that isn't something I've ever been and it wasn't something I was comfortable with being introduced for effect. I was keen they didn't add in blatantly untrue stuff and said so. They took it out straight away and I was both pleased and relieved. In my mind it was bad enough that my whole life was going to be put out there for everyone to see, without making me out to have problems I didn't have.

I'd go on to set when they needed me for press related matters, but for the most part I left them to it, although I did consult on riding styles and spent a lot of time with John Hurt. He was brilliant, such a genuine and lovely man. We got on really well and he was such a fantastic actor. To watch him was to watch a master at his art. I can't believe that in all of his career he never won an Oscar. I thought then and still do now, it was an honour to be portrayed by him. Mind you, he was a cheeky sod.

One day I was watching him and after a particular shot I said, "John you're not playing that like me, I'm not that nice."

He looked at me sardonically and in his gentle voice said, "Bob, if I played this part like you, no one would come watch the movie." Then he meandered away, giving me a wry smile over his shoulder as he left. So that was me told. I guess he might have had a point!

It's such a tragedy that cancer took him, but I was fortunate to be able to attend his funeral and pay my respects with so many of us who admired him a great deal.

Terry Biddlecombe, my old friend and a former three-times Champion Jockey, was also very friendly with John Hurt and because of that the movie company decided to use him as the on-set adviser for the technical aspects of racing. This worked out really well as it left me as the 'PR' man and meant that I wasn't needed on set all the time.

Over the years people have asked if I'm the one doing the actual riding in the movie, but the only footage of me is the bit of the original Grand National coverage that is blended into the film. The riders for the rest of it were John Burke, who'd won a National on Rag Trade and John Hatch, both of whom were the same size as John Hurt. They would do all the necessary stunt double work for him as there was no way I could have been matched as John's double. Not at my size! Of course the real star of the show, Aldaniti, played himself and was a natural for the camera.

I was quite happy being in the background. Starring in a film wasn't something I wanted. People might find that strange but it simply wasn't something I'd have considered. Until I won the National I had no real idea about fame or handling the limelight and even giving interviews made me nervous as hell. I had to develop a lot of resilience and an ability to hide my nerves really quickly, because once the movie came out I was warned by the film's producers that there was going to be a lot of publicity work. I was going to be even hotter property than I had been after the race. I figured they were exaggerating. I was wrong. If anything they had underestimated the amount of press work I was going to end up doing. In fact the true magnitude of it was hard to grasp and I certainly hadn't considered how far-flung it would be.

But they had to finish filming it first and I've got to admit, what with the actors being so true to their characters and the script writer listening to any objections I had, I'd say that the movie was 95% truth and 5% truth glamorised, which, when compared to a lot of other supposedly 'true stories' was fantastic. I think I got off really well.

There was one small thing that bothered me, the scene with the horseshoe. Two of my closest friends are Sally and Nigel Dimmer. Nigel was a jeweller who produced the Cheltenham Gold Cup and after my recovery, he'd had a silver horseshoe commissioned for me. In those days at Aintree there was a large board outside the weighing rooms and well-wishers or family and friends would pin telegrams and letters for you. On the day of the National I received so many moving telegrams, including a few from cancer patients, but the horseshoe was so very special and I did indeed slip it into my boot. Following the race I had it made into a necklace and gave it to Jo. I often thought about what happened to it as it's something that meant a great deal to me and I'm sorry I no longer have it. However, I guess it was more romantic within the movie for Jo to give it to me in the hospital. Like I said, truth glamorised and better a gift from the wrong source, than me being a drunk. At least I still have the very enduring friendship of Sally and Nigel, more about them later.

All in all, from the first contact about the prospect of a movie, to the script being finalised, the actors coming on board, through the actual filming process, all the way to the release, the whole thing took thirty-five months. A month before the final release date, I was told I could go and see a first screening with Lord Grade. The night before that I didn't sleep a wink. I was petrified.

You see, it's one thing to have been on set and watch scenes filmed, but you don't really get a feel for the movie as a whole. It's not done in sequence so all the scenes are disjointed and jumbled. John had advised me not to see the rushes as he said that they would really mess my head up. So it was just me and Lord Grade that saw the first version. It was originally 140 minutes long, but in those days anything over 123 minutes meant you had to have an intermission. We felt that it would spoil the flow of the movie to have a loo break and so it was reduced to an acceptable 106 minutes. It's a shame really as they cut out a few good bits but I know that it made sense to do it that way. Nowadays you'd get a 'director's cut' released on DVD but alas I'm sure whatever was cut out of Champions went into a big dustbin at the studio.

Later, when I got to see the final version of the movie, I was both delighted and relieved. They had gotten it right and John Hurt had done an amazing job. Very few people remember that he had lost his partner of fifteen years, the French model, Marie-Lise Volpeliere-Pierrot, in a riding accident in the January of 1983. The same accident had left John injured, yet he bravely continued to film and always said that he played the role for her. By the time filming ended he'd actually improved as a rider and I was chuffed watching him.

On the run up to the release it seemed like I was continually in demand. To this day I couldn't tell you how many interviews I took whilst promoting the movie, but it seemed to be non-stop. On occasion, I would think the interviewer was having a strange lapse in memory as they asked me the same question again, only to realise it wasn't them that had asked it, but the previous reporter. I was in a continual déjà vu loop.

This constant arc of publicity was just one of the new things I had to learn and in comparison, it was easy. My hardest struggle was becoming used to talking about myself and specifically about the indignity of cancer. That's not something many people talk about, indignity. The fact that cancer robs you of everything, your strength, your health, your looks and at times your mind, is not something most wish to recall. To make a habit of remembering it and to discuss it on an almost daily basis took its toll. My psyche was recoiling from the memories. I wanted to forget it, to bury it but that wasn't to be and the reason it couldn't be was the driving force behind all of that year and all of the subsequent publicity in my life. If the cancer taught me anything it was that I had a responsibility to all of those people that cared for and supported me. If recounting and reliving my story could help just one person, then it was something I needed to do.

φ

Being the face of a movie and attending premiers gives you a whole new appreciation of what actors have to go through for each and every movie they make. I only had to do it the once and it was exhausting. That might sound a little 'lovey', like I'm trying to compare the hardships of standing about doing press junkets and flying all over the world with the likes of going down the Skinningrove mines and of course, it isn't a fair comparison and I know which I'd rather do, but nonetheless, a movie launch is truly exhausting. I was knackered.

Alongside becoming the accomplished interviewee, and boy did I become good at press conferences and answering questions, I did have one constant thought; what on earth was I doing here? No, I'm not being modest, but to this day I still can't understand why anyone was that interested in my story. I'm serious. I mean I was hardly that famous, but I guess the only explanation is that we hit a 'sweet-spot' of public interest. The early eighties were full of hard luck stories and quite a bit of social unrest. I suppose Aldaniti and I were a tale of survival and we certainly had the best of happy endings. It had that feel-good factor and of course, horses.

I think every movie I've ever seen about horses seems to do okay. Even the dire attempts that have been released find an audience. Whatever the reason, *Champions* was taken to the public's heart and I'm incredibly glad and humbled that people were so swept up by it all. That was certainly the upside. As I've said, one of the downsides was being asked the same questions over and over and by now I would often go into auto-pilot, especially in the later months of the promotional tours, when I'd travelled a lot. Mind you, there'd be that one interviewer that would ask you something completely random in the hopes of catching you out. I used to like those, it was nice to be made to think.

If I thought all of it had been quite something up to this point, I had no clue what I was about to experience. A real life movie premier. Actually, a real life movie premier, with Royalty in attendance. I literally had to pinch myself as I arrived in London's Leicester Square, on the 1st March 1984. It's one of the most surreal moments in my life.

I'd seen coverage of these types of things on the TV before, but here I was, a guest of honour on a red carpet. We arrived in black cabs at the same time as John Hurt. I had my Mum and Dad and Jo with me. My Mum looked so glamorous next to my Father, who himself was fantastically smart and standing ramrod straight like the old soldier he was. I could see he was so proud of what had been achieved.

There were of course other family and friends attending including Mary and Richard, Howard Thompson, his partner Tina and of course my second mum, Howard and Derek's Mum, Mrs Thompson.

Howard recalls, *"It was an incredible feeling to be walking up the red carpet with cameras flashing at you and people wondering who you were. I kept hoping someone might ask me for my autograph! Alas they didn't, but they did Bob's."*

Flashes from a hundred cameras, people applauding, me being asked to sign autographs in amongst so many celebrities. The whole thing could have been terribly overwhelming if I hadn't had such a good relationship with the cast. They were old hands at this sort of thing and looked after me, making sure I knew where to be and ensuring I didn't mess up. It was great, really fun and the thing I remember most is everyone was smiling. Everyone. Even me! Not some forced smile either, I was genuinely pleased and happy that the film had been made. How could you not be thrilled that all these people had taken the time to tell your story? Add to that I was alive, the cancer that had threatened to kill me was gone and all the faces surrounding me were happy and thrilled to be there. It was a remarkable atmosphere and an amazing evening. One of the best in my life and I hadn't even made it into the cinema yet. I remember thinking, 'Wow, this is bigger than I thought it would be.'

When we got inside, it got bigger. We all had to line up ready to greet Her Majesty the Queen Mother. What an absolute honour that was! Can you imagine the Queen Mum watching a movie about you? That bit was a blur. I remember her chatting, but to be honest I can't really remember what we talked about. I think I asked her about one of her horses that had run that day and I'm sure to her any chat about racing and horses was welcome, as it saved her from trying to make polite small talk with me. After all, that's something I am really no good at.

After that highlight, we made our way into the cinema, found our seats, and I'm chuffed to say we weren't all stuck at the back, then the lights went down and out onto the stage stepped Shirley Bassey to sing the theme song, 'Sometimes'. Dame Shirley as she is now, live singing the theme song of the movie of my life. Ha! Yes, occasionally I do have to remind myself that this actually happened. But it did.

My goodness, Dame Shirley had a fantastic voice that night, although I have to say that I think Elaine Page did an even better job on the recording. Then it was time for the movie.

Now, I've been to many a movie, but I can't recall being nervous before the start of any of them. Well, not until this night. I was a bundle of tension. What if it wasn't well received by the audience? Worse still, what if my family were embarrassed? What if they thought I'd made a fool of myself? Fortunately none of that turned out to be the case, but as the opening titles appeared on screen I wasn't to know and I sat with my stomach churning, hardly seeing what was on the screen.

In the dark I waited and hoped and then, at the first emotional point in the movie there was an audible gasp from the audience. Later there were more. Laughs in the right places, sighs in the right places. It sounded like they were enjoying it. I relaxed a little, but not much.

As the closing scene faded and the house lights began to come up, I heard something I'd not heard in a cinema before. The audience started to applaud. Not just a light pattering of politeness, but whole-hearted exuberant applause. I looked around. John Hurt was beaming, as was the rest of the cast and crew. Beside me, my Mum was so proud, she was nodding her head and had tears in her eyes. Mary was chuffed to death and even though we're tough Yorkshire folk we do have our emotional moments. Rarely, if ever, have I felt such an intense feeling as I felt at that moment. It was a mixture of love and contentment and being truly humbled that I had been so fortunate to have been spared to enjoy all of this. As the lights became brighter I looked around in astonishment to see so many people in tears. Maybe Lord Grade was right, perhaps people would be interested in my story. By then I'd already lived it a million times, interview after interview so I'd started to become a little complacent with what I'd achieved.

After the film I was inundated by reporters wanting more interviews and quotes to go with the positive reviews. I've looked back at press clippings from that night and from the other premiers, of which there were so many, and I still can't believe it was that big. We even had an 'aftershow' party. It was another opportunity to meet the right people and be seen with the stars. It was at this party that I fully realised how much of a figurehead I'd become. I was the face I suppose and it was a case of go here Bob, go there Bob. Dutifully, I went off and did as I was told. Mind you, the cast were being pulled in every direction as well. All in all it was a stunning experience, one I am so glad to have been a part of and something I will never forget.

I'm sure you are thinking that with all those stars gathered together, I must have some 'film gossip' to share, but I'm afraid that there was none to be had. No divas, no prima-donnas, no demands for changing rooms with buckets of ice or a thousand flowers. None of that. We all got on fantastically and for a short time they were an extended and much loved family.

After London, it was one premier straight after another. That's meant literally. The following night it began in Manchester, which was great, although it must be said, not quite as glamorous as the Leicester Square one. Then the next night we moved on to Scotland, then back to York, then over to Ireland. After that, it was like someone had challenged me to see how many air miles I could manage in as short a time as possible. I went to premiers all over Europe, Australia, China and Japan to name but a few. In twelve months, I was hardly ever home.

Derek remembers:

"I was on holiday the night of the London premier which was unheard of for me, so I went to a later screening in York. Bob was there to promote it as he was at all the major screenings. I'll never forget that we brought my son Alex, who'd just been born and Bob said, "You go in, I'll push Alex round York for a couple of hours." I said to him he couldn't as he had to be in there as the star of the show and he replied, "No, I've seen it already. I've seen it a few times." I was worried that people would want to see him there but he said he'd see them at the end. So he went off with Alex and met us outside after it had finished. Everyone came out and he chatted about the film. How many film stars do you know that would do that? He was just so unassuming! It certainly hadn't changed him."

I remember that night in York. It was a great diversion from having to sit through the film again. Don't get me wrong, I liked the movie, still do, but you can get too much of a good thing. Alex and I had a lovely little walk.

Saying that I was busy is true, but you can imagine just how busy John, Jan and the cast were. Not only did they have to promote this film, but they were off filming new projects. That's why I was mainly alone and did become the front man for the PR throughout the tour. Occasionally they would join me, which took the pressure off, but I learned to travel in comfortable clothes and have a suit ready to change into for when I landed. I also learned in those days how little sleep I could manage on, as I can't sleep when travelling, whether it's on planes or in cars and I'd be whisked straight off to interviews the minute we touched down. I am slightly ashamed to say that I slept through several viewings and often had to wake myself up as the credits were rolling!

The European premiers were great and I got to mingle with Royalty again in Belgium, Spain and Monaco. No matter what country, the Royals love their horses and so this was going to be a winner with them. There's a reason it's called the Sport of Kings.

The next massive moment was to be the US premiers. We launched in the States in April and although it was initially well received it really didn't do brilliantly well. That sounds terribly disappointing, but you have to look at it in context. As I've said before, the Americans just don't get jump racing like the rest of the world and added to that, we were up against a huge Spring Release list with some tremendous competition. I'm not sure many stories about a UK jockey that most of them had never heard of would have stood tall against the likes of Ghostbusters, Terminator, Gremlins and Indiana Jones to name a few, but we still had our premier and it was good to be back in America again. Hollywood didn't come calling for me to become their next poster boy and I guess that was probably for the best!

I flew out to Tokyo a few hours before my 36th birthday. It's an overnight flight and I'd gone to lay down to try and get some rest. For one of the few times on board a plane, I managed to drift off, before I was awoken on the stroke of midnight by Annie Lennox, Dave Stewart, the rest of the Eurythmics and the airline cabin staff all singing happy birthday to me! What a gift! Annie is a wonderfully warm and funny lady and to have her sing to me was stunning. I didn't even mind being woken up for it! I was also able to attend her concert in Tokyo as a birthday gift. I did then and still do sometimes wonder at just how lucky my life was in general.

Of course it wouldn't have been me if during that trip and others I didn't have a few hair-raising moments.

Japan really surprised me. I'm not sure why I hadn't known before, but I was amazed to see that they're so keen on betting. I mean super keen. They'd bet on two flies crawling up a window. They were also the most particular with regard to photos. Each of their papers and publications wanted their own photograph, so it seemed I spent an entire day riding around a makeshift course jumping fences, just so they had enough 'unique' pictures. I reckon I must have jumped over a thousand times.

That evening I almost came a complete cropper when my racing expertise was put on show. I was invited to a race meeting and of course, being 'the jockey of the moment' I was eagerly asked to pick my favourite. Now, I'm like most racing people and believe in the form guide as the bible of all things, but I hadn't had any opportunity to see any form guides for the next race. I had seen the horses in the Parade Ring though, so I said that I fancied the Grey I'd seen being led around. It was a gorgeous horse and had looked relaxed, toned and keen. So, without anything else to go on I recommended it as my pick. After the various translations, I was met with confused looks, mumbles and vaguely polite smiles. I decided to stick a few yen on it myself. That's when I saw the betting board and realised I'd just tipped the field's 100-1 rank outsider.

I inwardly cringed and felt like a bit of a fool as the race started and my dear old Grey meandered about at the back of the field. There it stayed, tracking all the rest of the runners, detached by a couple of lengths, until coming round into the home straight, when it suddenly decided that now would be a good time to find its pace. Passing one, then two, then all the rest it romped home to win! I received sage nods of approval from all of the entourage. Phew! My pride and reputation intact plus a few extra yen I hadn't counted on!

I flew straight home and as soon as I had landed at Heathrow, was whisked off to Docklands where Derek was hosting the Stunt Man Awards of Great Britain. I'm not quite sure why, but I'd said I would hand out an award. I got there on time, did my bit and then jumped in a helicopter to be flown to Kempton where I was riding in a 'Legends' race. Lucky for me I was riding a horse that Lester Piggott had ridden a few days before. I asked him for his advice and he said, "Jump it straight out the gates and you've won this." I did and he was right! From Tokyo to the winning post, via stunt men in Docklands. My feet were sometimes not touching the ground.

The following day I was back on a plane for more PR... This is what I mean when I say it was exhausting. There wasn't much glamour and no time to go sight-seeing. This was totally knackering.

In the summer of 1984, I flew to South Africa and whilst there had a different sort of incident. The one thing we did get to do was stay in really nice hotels. This time I had a suite with a separate sitting room and in the en-suite, a luxurious deep bath. I decided this was just what I needed and started running the water, adding some bubbles, but not knowing it was a Jacuzzi… Short on time for the next press interview, I left the bath filling whilst I nipped into the sitting room to talk to the journalists. As I was giving my now well-practised answers I could see the interviewer's faces looking more and more startled. I turned to see a wave of bubbles surging out into the bedroom. Trying to explain to the hotel staff why I had unleashed a Tsunami of froth into one of their best suites left me a bit red faced. I felt so terribly embarrassed and had to keep telling them I hadn't done it on purpose. I mean it was hardly the rebellious type of thing a rock star would have done.

That same evening I thought I'd take myself off for a walk around the town, just to see if I could get a feel for the place. I was over tired to be honest and couldn't sleep. Travelling to so many wonderful places had been great, but really I hadn't gotten a look at much of anything and not really managed to 'connect' to the countries I had visited. Why I decided that Johannesburg in the early 1980's was the place to go sight-seeing in the middle of the night is beyond me. I was naïve and I hadn't considered that the protests against apartheid were gaining traction and that I, being a white man alone, could have been in danger.

Let's just say that the people responsible for me on that trip were not impressed by my wandering antics! In all fairness I hadn't seen anything untoward, the people I met had all been very kind and it had been nice to get out and look around.

The next day I was kept firmly in line but we went off to the races with Sol Kersner, the South African business magnate. All of the Miss World girls were there and I have never seen so many beautiful women in one place, it was mind boggling. We then went down to Sun City which Sol owned and went out on a safari trip before taking part in some para-gliding. I found that last activity quite boring, just hanging there doing nothing. Then it was back to Sun City to see Shirley Bassey performing music from the film.

The Sun City venue would later become infamous on the Artists against Apartheid album, but when I was there it was the ultimate playground, the Las Vegas of South Africa. I'd probably have enjoyed it a lot more had I not been working and had to be on my best behaviour!

The year was flying by in a haze of airport lounges and hotel rooms. I've been asked if I had a glamorous time with my hours filled by beautiful women and day long parties. Oh, how I wish! It couldn't have been further from the truth and I rarely had a moment to myself.

Australia, though brilliant, really was bloody hard work. We flew out for the release in October 1984, so by this time I'd been promoting for seven months. Now I know this might sound silly, but you forget just how far away Australia is and how big it is until you have to get to it and around it in a few days! I seemed to spend an awful lot of time on planes. In Sydney, our flight arrived late and the TV film crew were waiting on the runway, I was filmed walking off the plane and then whisked straight off to the various TV stations. I know I didn't get to see any of that lovely country other than the inside of hotel rooms, airports and cinemas! One day I will get back to it for a proper look.

Before returning home from Australia I received a phone call from my secretary Jane to tell me that there were some financial irregularities in my bank that I needed to resolve as soon as possible. I didn't think too much about it. Probably just an errant bill. Sadly it was far from just a bill.

What I wasn't to know was that it was more than my bank account that had gone bust. It was my marriage too.

Some might say, "That was a wrap!"

The Odds-On
Favourite

Prior to having cancer I don't think I was overly altruistic. After all, I am the stereotypical, 'careful with pennies' Yorkshire man at heart. Yet I'd like to think I always helped out a friend or did what I could to support those in need. It's simply that I never thought that much past racing. Life had just been a constant battle of wasting, racing and healing, with of course the carousing that most people seem to remember me for in those early days. However, the cancer changed me in more ways than I realised. Not immediately, but quite quickly, I came to understand that I had a responsibility to those that had helped me live and to those still fighting.

Thus began the start of the Bob Champion Cancer Trust.

It shouldn't be a surprise to anyone that the British public is emotionally attached to sporting stories of endeavour and triumph, none greater than those that involve their national icons of sport. The consequences of this attachment to Aldaniti and myself were to become apparent very soon.

In the first few days following the '81 National the outpouring of generosity from the public was incredible. I had raced because I had something to prove to myself and to everyone suffering from cancer, but I never expected to be the focus of such unselfish financial sharing.

At first, people from all over the world, but especially the UK, sent their Grand National winnings to the Royal Marsden, care of me. From the smallest of successful wagers to some rather larger amounts, it seemed a nice spontaneous gesture and one that was certainly appreciated, but I didn't expect it to continue. I'm sure no one did. As the days went on and the donations kept coming, the doctors on the cancer wards called me up and suggested we should have a chat about what to do with the money. When they told me how many letters had been received in such a short amount of time, I felt overwhelmed in much the same way as I'd felt on winning the race itself. Even today, all these years later, it still fills me with emotion.

Looking back, it's easy to admit that we didn't really know what to do with the money. By the time the first wave of donations began to slow down there was several thousand pounds in the pot.

I met with Professor Michael Peckham (or to give him his full title, Sir Michael John Peckham FMedSci) and Nick Embiricos to discuss how the money should be used. Initially I thought we could perhaps brighten up a number of areas in the hospital. I could only give advice based on my direct experiences and whilst every member of the medical staff at the Royal Marsden was great, you did spend a great deal of time sitting around waiting. Some of the places you spent a lot of time in were fairly drab. I really believed and thankfully my gut instincts were to be borne out with later studies, that having the right aesthetic atmosphere can make a difference to the healing process. I didn't think it was rocket science.

You know yourself, that if you enter a hospital waiting room that's painted horribly and has no atmosphere you immediately feel worse and a bit depressed. Imagine how that affects the emotions of someone who is looking death in the face?

Added to that and probably due to my immediate desire to get fit again after my treatment, I thought there was a need for better physical rehabilitation. Having tried to get fit in the UK, I knew first-hand how hard it was. The weather doesn't help so you need somewhere that not only has the right equipment and atmosphere but with specialists that can help you mentally progress as well as physically. The two are so tightly interlinked. Often you feel that your body is letting you down, you know? Basically you become angry at yourself and this is a dangerous time when people are at their most vulnerable. It's then you need the physical and spiritual support of a professional physio.

So, at that first meeting, we decided that if we could, we should fund a 'makeover' of the physiotherapy, out-patients and rehabilitation centres. I felt that these areas within the hospital were vitally important and should receive financial support. However, our initial ideas soon became unrealistic.

Not because they were too ambitious, in fact completely the opposite. The donations hadn't stopped coming in. They had slowed from the initial wave, but they hadn't ceased. As we took our time drawing up the plans for the 'makeover' the money kept coming. We began to wonder just how big a makeover we could achieve. By 1983 we realised that we had received so much money that we had to do something much more formal. Another meeting was called.

The conversation was quick, decisive and there and then the Bob Champion Cancer Trust was born. That sounds very simplistic and I suppose it is, because it took a lot of help from a lot of people in the background, those who understood the technicalities of creating a charity and defining how the money should be allocated to make the reality of it happen. But nonetheless, it did happen quickly. Simply put, we hadn't expected to need a charity, so it all had to be arranged pretty sharpish.

I thought that if we were careful, prudent and considered, the money would last for a few years. I'm sure that Professor Peckham, Nick and all the rest expected the same, but as you will see the Trust developed a momentum that took it to far greater heights than we could ever have envisioned. But back in '83, I thought we should probably have a fund-raiser or two to keep the coffers topped up. It might also raise the interest levels in the Trust. I wasn't sure what the events would look like or how we would make them happen, but I figured I knew people, this new-found celebrity of mine meant I was in the public-eye and it certainly seemed the public were already on side.

I can chuckle about it now, but looking back to those early days of the Trust, there was no way, and I really mean no way, I'd ever have believed you that we'd still be going after all this time. It's knocking on for thirty-five years. That's incredible. I certainly know that I didn't really understand what we were achieving until we opened the first research centre. We didn't just give an existing building a lick of paint. We didn't just freshen up a physio or a gym. We not only created a better environment for patients but incredibly, we opened a full-blown research centre for the battle against cancer. That was when the enormity of it hit me. I was so proud of all those that had made it possible and I didn't think we could ever top that achievement. Of course I was happily proved wrong when the Trust opened its second research centre a few years later.

The leap from a bit of a 'makeover' to opening research centres is one that you may think takes some explaining, but it comes down to a simple premise. Had I been diagnosed with the type of cancer I had, only a year or two earlier, I would have died. It was only the pioneering work of scientists in the field of cancer treatment that had saved me. I felt, that if we really had enough money to do some work in that area then we should.

I had been cured of testicular cancer because of a new treatment involving the use of a drug called cis-platin. I was one of the first people in the UK to receive the new treatment and it was down to a man called Andrew Thomson. He'd made this discovery while working in the USA but then came to work at the University of East Anglia, (UEA) in Norwich. It's only quite recently that I learned how cis-platin (platinum) was discovered as a drug that could kill cancer cells.

In 1965 whilst working in the laboratory of Barnett Rosenberg with Loretta Van Camp and Eugene B. Grimley, Andrew was using platinum diodes to run electricity through bacteria cells in an effort to kill them by electrocution. What he observed and subsequently went on to prove was that it wasn't the electricity that killed them but the platinum. This was to be a major breakthrough and subsequently they injected platinum compounds into mice with sarcoma and showed that the cancer regressed. This was a break-through that I, along with many untold thousands, am profoundly grateful for. I only wish they could have done something about the smell! Today chemotherapy can be given in so many different ways, even tablets that can be taken at home. It's remarkable how so much has been achieved in such a relatively short space of time.

That advance in treatment through research prompted our idea of developing a charity devoted to improving methods of de-tecting and treating testicular, prostate and bladder cancers and, ul-timately, setting the goal of eradicating deaths from male cancers altogether. Can you imagine that? At the time of writing this, in late 2017, more than 250,000 people in the UK will be told they have cancer annually; 21,400 of these will be prostate cancer, a condi-tion that is predicted to overtake lung and breast cancer as the most commonly diagnosed variant in the UK by 2018. Testicular cancer rates have risen by 70% in the last 30 years. That's a lot of people who could be saved.

With the ambitious goal set, we knew we had to start being serious in our fund raising efforts. The first big idea was the Al-daniti Ball. It was a huge event in November 1984 and it raised a staggering £180,000 which in those days was a crazy amount of money. It was a Black-Tie event held at the Dorchester Hotel, with a champagne reception, an auction and then dancing. Not really the thing for a rural Yorkshire man but I was learning fast and didn't make too many faux pas.

The whole evening was actually a very simple format that worked very well and back in the mid-80's was the 'thing' to do. People with money were keen to 'see and be seen' doing the right thing. The auction itself was amazing. We had a nomination for future stud fees on three racehorses, one of which went for £25,000 alone.

We ran the balls every two years after that and they always attracted a big crowd. I say we, because by now the Trust needed some administrative support and thank goodness in 1986 we found Lucy Wilkinson. She has been our stalwart backbone since those early days and without her I doubt we would have achieved a tenth of what we have. Always looking after the details that I would certainly not think of, always thinking ahead and always inventive. In one of the early Aldaniti Balls she even managed to secure a donation of a car from Jaguar, which she then had to drive into the ballroom.

Over the years the format of the Balls began to go out of fashion and like all things, they had run their course. We held the last one in 2006. By then people were more understated about their charitable donations, but the Dorchester events were incredibly fun whilst they lasted although I never did learn how to dance.

Alongside them and the rest of the more usual charity events we staged, we also ensured we kept a focus on horse racing and horse related activities. It was, after all, how most people had heard about the Trust in the first place.

In 1985 Nick Embiricos came up with the idea for me to ride Aldaniti from Buckingham Palace to Aintree, arriving the day before the Grand National and ending with us making an appearance at the track. I thought it was brilliant concept and as a fund-raiser and profile-raiser it certainly was, but my goodness was there so much to arrange. The logistics of an event like that are huge and it needed so many people to become involved. You can't just saunter up half the length of Britain with a horse nowadays. Back in the 1600's I guess there were lots of coaching inns that you could stop at, with stables for the horse and a bed for the rider, but I'm not sure the average hotel would be equipped in the same way now, so it needed a lot of planning and support. We certainly couldn't have done any of it without the help from the British Horse Society. They were incredible with their assistance in providing us with routes and information, introductions to local vets and a host of other things, all of which, including their time, they donated freely.

Our goal was to get a relay of riders and for them to raise sponsorship of £1,000 per mile. That was a huge ask in 1985, but so many people came forward I was immediately encouraged that it was achievable. Initially we advertised in the 'Horse & Hounds' and various other racing journals, magazines and papers. We asked the Royal Marsden to contact cancer patients past and present and our trustees spread the word in the business world in London. Of course, this was all pre-Internet and social media, but by good old-fashioned phone calls and letters and personal meetings, we managed to get people involved.

With perhaps the exception of some of the celebrities, everyone that took part had in some way been touched by cancer. Whether they were riding for their mother, father, brother, sister or themselves, each had a story and an emotional connection to the walk. It was so humbling to see, talk to and be a part of their lives, even if only for a mile. Some people were quite poorly and others, well it had given them something to look forward to, that all important 'hope' that you need in order to get through the ordeal that is cancer treatment. Many of our sponsored riders had done incredible things to raise the money, including school children who were determined to be part of it. I think the vast majority of riders raised more than the £1,000 we'd set as the target.

We started out on 1st March 1987. The Queen had graciously allowed us to begin at Buckingham Palace. That walk north to Liverpool was to bring us face to face with the very worst of British weather and the first day was no exception. It was bitterly cold, yet it was with immense pride that I watched the great jockey, Jonjo O'Neill, himself suffering from cancer and in the middle of his treatment, start proceedings dressed in the blue and white colours of Nick Embiricos and sat atop Aldaniti. Jonjo was not well, but like I had been, he was determined not to be beaten. I'm so pleased to see that he has gone from strength to strength since. Dick Stowe, who suffered from Motor Neurons disease also rode on that first day, another charity that Josh Gifford was keen to support after one of his stable lads had been diagnosed with it at an early age.

We had some very familiar faces with us including Princess Anne and Fergie (as she was then, now of course Sarah, the Duchess of York), as well as celebrities such as Bob Hoskins, Lindsey de Paul, Michael Aspel and the lovely Alison Steadman. Of course John Hurt was there too and as usual, he was brilliant.

We were in the middle of nowhere in this tiny village one day when he realised he needed to use a toilet and a simple hedge wasn't going to cut it. He went up and knocked on the nearest front door. The lady who opened it looked flabbergasted as John Hurt asked if he could use her loo! Lucy remembers the look of amazement on her face that was still there when he thanked her on the way back out and jumped up on the horse! Can you imagine John Hurt standing on your doorstep? He was great fun and he always said that he thought Aldaniti recognised him. I'm sure he was right.

Because we kept off the main highways and went through small villages we'd have people running out of their houses to give us money and we constantly needed two or three people walking alongside us with buckets. Whether it was 50p or £10 the general public were unfailing in their generosity. It was an incredible event. Due to the kindness of the public we didn't have to use any of the money raised in sponsorship to cover the costs and it all went into the charity fund.

Like I said, you just don't realise what's needed to make an event like that happen. Added to the stables for the horses each and every night, you also need accommodation for the riders, which often was someone's sofa or spare room. Usually there were five or so of us sharing. In fact, now I come to think of it, the horses were much better accommodated than we were.

We also needed to have a vet on standby within each area, supplies of feed, water, somewhere to dry out blankets, prepare the tack and so on and so on. Some of these villages were so remote it must have looked like they were being invaded. There were Land Rovers and horse boxes parked up, people arriving and being picked up when we did the changeovers and of course the medical care for the poorly and disabled riders.

On the night before we arrived at Aintree I became aware of a problem. Since the cancer treatment I'd started suffering with gout. Now anyone who's ever had it will know the immense pain it causes and I had a flare up. It was in my big toes and my feet were so swollen I couldn't get my shoes on. The next day I needed to be in riding silks and boots. I was swallowing Allopurinol and every 'herbal' gout concoction they could throw at me, but nothing was working. The next morning I was still in agony but I suppose the one thing I am fairly sure of about myself is that I ain't a quitter and I won't let people down. I can't tell you the agony I was in as I pulled those boots on. It could have been ten times worse and still have been worth every moment as I rode Aldaniti around the Parade Ring and in front of the Aintree stands. We had completed a distance of 225miles, had a marvellous time sharing the experience with all those that helped us and, not insignificantly, raised just shy of one million pounds.

φ

In those first few years we had raised so much more money than we could ever have imagined. That early notion of sprucing up buildings had long been surpassed by the idea of funding research, but it was Professor Peckham who first suggested an actual bricks and mortar research centre. I can remember the emotions sweeping through me when he did. To raise money for investigations into treatments was one thing, but to raise money for a dedicated facility that could make a real difference and have a lasting legacy was something else entirely. I felt a drive and a desire to achieve that as strongly as I felt the drive and desire to ride winning racehorses. It was quite the moment.

In 1986 the Bob Champion Cancer Research Unit within the Royal Marsden NHS Trust Hospital at Sutton, Surrey was opened. What an amazing achievement, I was totally in awe of what we'd accomplished and never in a million years did I think I would put my name to a building such as that. Thinking back to those dark days of chemo, I'd barely managed to fight through it and yet here I was looking at the forefront of technology aimed at eradicating the very thing that nearly killed me. It has, since that day to this, been my absolute privilege to work with and know some of the most brilliant minds in cancer research. Their skill and dedication is inspiring.

The Trust was certainly established now and for the next 10 years we were to have many more events like the inaugural 'Aldaniti Walk' and not just from London to Liverpool.

A trip to Ireland in 1990 saw us all on tour for The Irish Roadshow. This was in conjunction with the Irish Cancer Society. I've always loved travelling across to Ireland and on this trip we were to walk to many of the racecourses. Now, it is a significant understatement to say the Irish like their horses. I'm not sure there's a society anywhere in the world where the average person in the street loves horses as much. The whole nation seems to have some sort of affinity with them and of course, they love their horse racing and especially sending their horses over to try to take England's top racing honours, be it on the flat or especially over the jumps. The Cheltenham Festival is the pinnacle of this friendly rivalry and it annually plays host to tens of thousands of Irish fans every March in the week of St Patrick's Day. With a Guinness tent the size of a football pitch the 'craic' as they would say is mighty. Of course their horse breeding programs are also exceptional and over the years they have produced some outstanding chasers, including the best of them all, Arkle. Or as he was known by the whole of the Irish nation, 'Himself'. So it was a racing certainty that we would get a warm and affectionate welcome and sure enough we did.

As with the Aldaniti Walk and all the later walks and rides, we were relying on the generosity of the public and equine societies to provide horses, vets and places for us to sleep. Not that we would have needed to worry, for as well as their love of horses, the Irish have a definite sense for hospitality. If anything, they might just be a little too hospitable, and I'm not sure anyone on that beautiful island knows how to pour a small drink for their guests. On one memorable night, Lucy may have drunk more than was good for her and, once behind the wheel, realised that she was in no fit state to drive. She decided to pull over and park, but instead careered over a little bridge on just two wheels and a little more Dutch courage than I think she was used to! I'm pretty sure that had she been perfectly sober, she'd never have taken the bridge as quickly or perhaps as well as she did! The Irish police, An Garda Síochána, however were less than amused and I watched in horror as they pulled up beside her. The guard stepped up to her window and I don't know to this day what she said to them but perhaps she managed to throw a little of their own charm back at them. By promising not to drive again that night, she was let off with a warning.

Thank goodness as I'm not sure any of us would have bailed her out! Of course it gives me great pleasure to remind her of it, often!

We rode to Cork for a point-to-point meeting and I recall cantering up to the winning post as two kids aged about seven or eight, rode up to the steeplechase jumps. They were on 12-hand ponies yet had no fear in taking the fences. One of the boys stood out, just in the way he was handling the pony. It's like watching a good dancer or a good football player. You don't have to see 'it' for long and you may not even be able to say what 'it' actually is, but there's a spark that sets the talented apart. This young fellow had it. I thought to myself, 'One day, young man, you are going to be a great jockey.' I later found out his name and tucked it away in my memory. About ten or twelve years later, sure enough Wayne Lordan began to make his mark as a flat jockey. He continues to have a great career and was recently taken on by Aidan O'Brien. In May of 2017, Wayne won his first Classic, taking out the 1,000 Guineas on the filly, Winter. Just goes to show that natural talent prevails.

Later during that trip, I was asked to take part in a pro-celebrity golf tournament and was partnered up with the snooker player Willie Thorne. I'm glad Willie was such a generous and humorous personality, for I could jump hurdles with the best of them, but golf? I'm afraid to say it's not my game and I didn't succeed in much more than making it round the course. Gladly, I can't recall my score but I'm sure if you asked Willie what his handicap was, he'd have said me.

That trip, like all of our trips raised the awareness of the Trust as well as a lot of money, but it was subtly different in that somehow it seemed more relaxed than many of the other ones we did. Perhaps it was down to this strange affinity the Irish have with horses, or that no one was in a rush when we were coming through their towns and villages. The traffic didn't try and run you off the road and everyone would take the time out to say hello and to pat the horses. It also seemed they were all so knowledgeable about racing in general and so the conversations you could have were in depth and always fun. Of course, I told anyone that would listen that English horses were the better jumpers and I got good natured laughs and knowing looks thrown back at me. I'm not sure I managed to convince many that I was right, but it was certainly fun trying. As if to emphasise the fact that I might have overlooked a thing or two, our route took us near to the magnificent Coolmore Stud, in County Tipperary. Founded by the original O'Brien genius, Vincent, it is headquarters to the world's largest breeding operation of thoroughbreds and has, through its racing arm in Ballydoyle, raced some significant champion horses.

We were over in Ireland for 10 days and it was with mixed feelings I left because the pace of life was so much more relaxed and as fund raising events go, it was certainly much less demanding. However, my liver and I think Lucy's was relieved to be going home.

In 1992 we opened the Aldaniti Rehabilitation Unit and The Bob Champion Lounge at the Royal Marsden Hospital. This is a special leisure area for those requiring long term in-patient care. It was the realisation of what I had long thought, it's so important for rehabilitation that patients feel comfortable and relaxed whilst receiving treatment.

Of course riding in the charity events sometimes required me to lose a little of my more substantial frame. For a flat race at Aintree in 1995 I had to shed over 2st and I can tell you it was hell. So much harder than it had been in my racing days as I was completely out of practice and used to eating what I liked. At first when Nick suggested it I thought it was a great idea but as the weeks wore on I was miserable and hungry. Of course there wasn't a chance in hell that I wasn't going to be capable of racing, but my God what an enormous effort that took. I made the weight on the day and took the field beside nine truly legendary jockeys. I'd like to say that I won but it was a close thing and I actually came in second to Maurice Barnes. It was amazing to be back in the saddle and racing at Aintree, even though none of us were fit enough or young enough to jump, there was still an atmosphere and camaraderie that you don't get anywhere else. We all had a laugh and whilst it was for a good cause we all also wanted to win. There were lots of jokes about excess weight, but I think on that day we'd all done ourselves proud and the crowd loved it.

In 1996 we agreed to the massive undertaking of 'The Ride for Life' that would see us go from Holyrood Palace in Edinburgh to Buckingham Palace, London. We challenged ourselves to raise £1M to go towards a research lab at the Royal Marsden, knowing that if we raised it, the Institute of Cancer Research would match us in funding.

Again it required a huge amount of preparation and this time I would need a different horse, because my old friend Aldaniti wasn't up to walking the whole way. He'd start us off and be there again for the finish, but that was as much as he could manage.

We invited people to sponsor us, ride with us or offer their horse for me to ride. I knew this was going to be a challenge for me too, as it was 600miles and I'd be in the saddle for up to eight hours each day. I've got to say that the Pony Club was incredible. They supplied horses where needed and helped us out as much as they could. The hunts all had horses for us and they were marvellous too. Without the help of the equine industry none of the walks we did would have been possible.

The night before the start, I got to stay at Holyrood Palace. I did wonder how a Yorkshire boy who could so easily have ended up down the mines, ended up in a palace. It was fabulous. Janette and I really did feel like royalty. They don't make buildings like that anymore. The walls are so thick and everything about it is so substantial. Mind you I was glad it was summer as I imagine it could be a bit draughty and chilly in winter. The beds were huge and really soft. I know Janette thoroughly enjoyed her stay and felt like a queen. It was a shame we were only able to stay the one night. All the Trust team and supporters got together and had dinner that evening, it was to be the last luxury for some time. With all of these events we have such a great crew, and it's a laugh even though it's bloody hard work. To be fair I knew that I had the easy job, because all I had to do was sit on the horse all day being polite to people. I had none of the worry about the logistics. That said, it was hard going on my bum!

Unlike the first walk, this time we began on a beautiful sunny morning. Aldaniti was in fine form and with a police escort I felt amazing, well except for one thing. Some idiot had decided that it would be a great idea for me to wear a kilt. I've got to say I felt so embarrassed and I'm certainly not one for wearing 'skirts' no matter what David Beckham might suggest. Before you ask, yes I did wear pants underneath, it was bad enough that the saddle leather chafed my thighs without adding anything else to the mix. I'm glad I'm not a woman as their legs must get really quite chilly! One Scottish journalist commented that the kilt was off before you could say, 'Hoots Mon' and he wasn't wrong, although I kept it on long enough for the grand parade as we rode out and the walk officially started.

I can honestly say that this was a brilliant event and that I met some absolutely wonderful people. It was a very hot summer which meant the turn out along the route was fantastic, but the heat did lead to difficulties of its own. You'd think it would be easier if the weather was nice but we had to be careful of the horses and it was harder to ride in the heat. As one of my ambitions since being a little boy was to be a cowboy in the wild west, I gritted my teeth and imagined being on the dusty plains. Several people joined us on endurance rides and stuck with us for some distance. I got the chance to get to know them and their company made all the difference. It's lovely meeting new people and hearing their stories. Often people rode with us because they or a family member had been through cancer. Having their companionship on the walk was exceptional. I was humbled by their effort in joining us and pleased that they felt it was so worthwhile.

In the evenings all we really wanted to do was to drop into bed, but everywhere we stayed had arranged a charity night, be it a hotel or someone's home there was something happening in the evening and we'd have to be involved. Don't get me wrong, we didn't begrudge a moment of it, but you can imagine how tired everyone was, particularly as we were up until 1am most nights.

Now we had asked people to supply horses for the event and we ran all of the checks that we could to ensure that they were suitable. But... As we might say in Yorkshire, 'There's nowt so queer as folk' and you just can't legislate for how some people think. Of all the horses we have ever been loaned, we had three that stick in my mind for all the wrong reasons.

First off was a horse that hadn't been broken in. Can you imagine how dangerous that was on the roads? He reared up, charged off and nearly caused a pile up. I thought I could hold him, but he threw me and I went down hard on my knee. It was incredibly painful and I knew it was going to be an issue for the rest of the ride. The owners had been adamant that he was broken in and safe to ride. What utter rubbish.

Next came a great big yolk of a horse, totally nuts! I could sense he was going to be a handful as he was all over the place. I saw a ploughed field next to me so I took him off in there to calm him down and wear him out. I thought I'd gallop him until he dropped. It didn't work and just holding him on the road was a nightmare which hurt my knee even more. To make matters worse we'd taken a wrong turn and had to walk along a busy A-road. I know I was fuming and I'm ashamed to say I took it out on one of our young volunteers who was helping organise the walk. I know I shouted at her, yelling that it was her fault. It wasn't of course, but I was in pain and becoming more and more frustrated.

Besides Mary, Lucy is one of the only people who gets away with telling me off. We've worked together for almost thirty years now on the charity and she knows my moods. We'd have very lively 'discussions' behind bushes or she would take me off to one of the horse boxes and yell at me to stop yelling in front of the public if I got too cross. It's funny looking back, but I know she was right. I like to think that I'm an angel but I'm honest enough to admit that I'm not and I do often lose my temper. As with the old days of racing though, I calm down quickly and it's usually a storm in a teacup. Being a man I don't always think of the consequences and I once snapped at Lucy in front of a little girl riding with us. Lucy, completely justified, gave me a right going over for upsetting the child. I hadn't realised she'd get upset just because I was cross with someone else. Lucy always blames me when things go wrong and says it's because I'm not where I should be, but I think this is just rubbish. Although I probably wouldn't tell her that.

I do know that when I get mad it's usually because I'm angry at myself and not the other person, it just doesn't come out that way.

During the walk we went through some lovely towns, and you see so much more going slowly on horseback. You have the time to notice the greens and pubs, the churches and houses. We travelled down through the Borders then through Newcastle, York, Sheffield, Derby, Coventry, Stratford and Oxford, avoiding all the main routes. Often though we'd have to cross a motorway via one of their bridges. I hated this. I'm not sure if it was a dream or a random thought I'd had, but I know I was petrified that if the horse bolted I'd be over the bridge and into motorway traffic. It terrified me and I did think that perhaps I would land safely in a lorry filled with water and fishes going under the bridge. The weird things you think about on a 600mile walk!

On one of the last days, as we were coming in towards London, I was on a lovely little horse. She was very pleasant and such a pleasure to ride so it was such a shame that I had to swap to a big horse that I really didn't like the look of. As a jockey you come to have an instinct and I knew that there was something wrong with this one as it came out of the box. Against better judgement I mounted him and we cantered around the indoor school where we'd stopped to do the swap over. He seemed ok, just a little feisty but I was still wary. I should have trusted my instincts. This was to be problem horse number three. We left the school and he bolted, took off at a gallop straight across a main road. He was full on and nothing was stopping him, well nothing until he came to a ditch, which is where he ended, upside down with me on top of him pretty bashed up. I decided there and then I wasn't riding him again and certainly he wasn't fit to take into London, so it was back to the little mare I'd been on before.

Then I was reunited with the old boy and together Aldaniti and I rode through London on the 5th August. This day will stay with me always. I remember looking at the buildings as we rode through Piccadilly, Regents Street and Oxford Circus and being amazed at how beautiful some of them were. You don't see the beauty when you are in a car or bustling through the streets normally. We of course had a police escort and they had arranged for all the traffic lights to be on green as we approached them. We were led into the Mall by a Scottish piper and beside me was Tracey Bailey on Mr Frisk, the horse who recorded the fastest time ever to win a Grand National. He wasn't always the most calm of rides but on that day he was impeccably behaved and to add a bit more ceremony, we were given a 'guard of honour' by the Grace Sisters, with their polo sticks raised in the air as we came into the Mall.

We were actually early for our reception with Her Majesty the Queen so we did have to wait for a short time. Whilst we were standing outside the Palace, the Queen Mother drove out and did a double turn around the Victoria Memorial roundabout so that she could get a second look at us. I know she would have loved seeing all of the horses there and indeed she gave us a friendly wave on her way out.

We met the Queen and Aldaniti famously spat her carrot back out at her, he just wasn't up for carrots. Had it been a mint he'd definitely have had it. He had a thing for Polos and in fact that was the reason his groom, Wilf lost £1,000. Rowntree's at the time had been running a competition, like something out of Willy Wonka, and had put a number of gold mints into special packets. Wilf thought it had just been in his pocket too long and become discoloured. Rather than holding it in his mouth the way he would normally, he simply gave it to Aldaniti. It wasn't until he recounted it to his wife, Beryl, that he realised his mistake!

After we had met Her Majesty we attended a canapés and champagne reception. We'd finished our longest ride to date, I was absolutely shattered but it was worth every step, bump and moment of lost sleep. In the end we sadly had fallen short of the £1M but still it brought us one step closer to the research centre.

ф

I've told you already, I'm at heart a shy person and I still am, despite all the years appearing in front of cameras. Yes, I can cope with it, but I found TV shows initially quite daunting. In the busy years following the National I must have appeared on most of the popular variety or quiz shows and I did wonder that people weren't sick of seeing me. However, I went on them for the sake of the

Trust and got through the majority without too many problems, but it was rare for me to really enjoy them. One that was different, an awful lot of fun and one of the best experiences I've had, was the 1997 Christmas special of Gladiators.

It was a great laugh, but bloody hard work! The program producers reckoned it would be good to pit a team of jockey's versus television celebrities. On our side was Peter Scudamore, Tony Dobbin, Carl Llewellyn and Willie Carson. Thing is, I think people underestimate just how fit jockeys have to be. In America they say that jockeys are the fittest athletes in the world and it was interesting to see the response to us taking on Mr Motivator! Especially given Willie, Peter and myself were already 'retired'.

You don't realise how much goes into it, we started practising at 6am and had eight hours of it before filming began in front of a live audience. We were knackered before we started! Compared to the Gladiators, Willie was tiny. What a spectacle.

By the end of it we were nineteen points ahead and had hammered the celebs. More than hammered, we'd absolutely smashed them, including Mr Motivator. The way it works is we could have used the points to have a 9.5 second time advantage over them for the last race, 'The Eliminator' but we thought we'd do the decent thing and start off at the same time.

This final race is a relay and as I was the captain for our team it was down to me to run the last obstacle, the Travelator. It's the equivalent of running flat-out up an escalator. Well I thought I'd practice it during the day and could I get up there? Not a chance. I tried for a quarter of an hour and still couldn't do it. I thought, 'This is going to be horrendous tonight!' In frustration I said to the chap running it, "What am I doing wrong?"

"You'll never get up it in a million years mate, you're looking at it!"

I said, "Why didn't you tell me that before?"

"You didn't ask, but now you have, you've just got to look above it."

I did that and ran straight up it! Just to make sure, I did it another six times to be certain.

On the night I got up it with no problem and we won by over five seconds, despite starting even. None of us had realised just how much hard work it was going to be and I certainly wasn't at my fittest. Still it was great fun and we raised £5,000 that night.

Of course it's not all been about having fun at events or on TV, there is a very serious side to what we do in the Trust. The money we raised that night was added to the pot for the research centres.

In 2000 we opened The Bob Champion Research Centre for Urological Cancers in conjunction with the Institute of Cancer Research. It was the first male dedicated cancer research facility in Europe. You can imagine how proud I was of this as there has always been a bit of a stigma attached to male cancer. I think mainly because men don't like talking about their problems and are very reluctant to get things checked. I'm a prime example of that. Personally I think any cancer research is critical but some of the cancer campaigns and charities do get a lot more coverage on the television and in the community. I don't begrudge them it at all, but for male cancers it does tend to be still a little hush-hush.

In 2001 we received the amazing news that the researchers had gone as far as they could with testicular cancer research and that the statistics had changed from a 27% survival rate when I was diagnosed to a fantastic 95%. It was at this point that we made the decision to transfer funding to prostate cancer. Many people have asked me why I didn't just bring the Trust to an end having done my bit? The thing is, the Trust is more than me. It always was more than me and it certainly is now. There are so many dedicated people involved and to stop was never an option. We always make sure that we have enough money to carry on funding the dedicated projects for at least several years.

The reason for moving to prostate cancer research was that testicular cancer was considered 'cured' while prostate cancer was badly funded and dramatically under researched. Professor Colin S. Cooper is a leading cancer researcher who is currently Professor of Cancer Genetics at Norwich Medical School. He explained to me that in 2001 there was only five pence per man spent on prostate cancer research. Five pence! That seemed ridiculous and something that we could definitely change. Professor Cooper went on to become involved in a National Institute of Cancer Research, Prostate Cancer Collaborative Forum from 2001 to 2011 which included the Department of Health, the Medical Research Council and Cancer Research UK. It was to tackle the gross underfunding of male cancer research. I like to think that our Trust's change of direction was instrumental in creating a seed change in the minds of the bigger charities when it came to funding.

With the change in direction came the need to continue and indeed, increase, our fund raising activities. Unless you are a nationally significant charity, like the Poppy Appeal, or the Wings Appeal, that takes place at the same time each year, you have to continue to be innovative. The truth of the matter is that fund raising for any charity, even the big national ones, can become very monotonous, and monotony is a real danger if you are trying to get people to put their hands in their pockets. So it was that in 2010 I decided it would be great to do something different. Something that wasn't another ball or another walk.

I can remember coming up with this idea of '60:60', a joint venture with the Injured Jockeys Fund. I'd visit all 60 racecourses in Britain in 60 consecutive days, which sounds easy, but it's not! The plan was I would drive to each venue criss-crossing the country in a 17,000mile marathon. Each course had to have a race meeting on the day of the visit, and people could buy packages to come and join me. In addition, on each day, in return for a £50 minimum donation, anybody could gain free entry to the club enclosure of their chosen meeting, discover how racing works behind the scenes, meet me and walk the track before racing started. There would also be opportunities for a photo with the jockeys and visiting celebrities as well as a prize draw.

As the planning kicked in I'd be waking up in the middle of the night trying to rearrange races in my head. Thankfully, Lotus, the luxury sports car manufacturer, decided to sponsor us. It seemed like a great idea. In the run up they sent one of their test drivers who took me out on country lanes doing 90mph. I was petrified!

You never knew if a tractor was going to be around the next bend and I can honestly admit to it being one of the things that has truly scared me in my life. You'd think a man that rides fast horses over enormous jumps would be able to handle anything at speed, but not this. Maybe it's a control thing, but going out with that type of driver is not something I'd like to repeat. I did get the opportunity to take the Lotus Evora out on the test track and that was definitely okay.

We set off on Sunday the 18th April at Ascot and concluded by returning to Ascot on Wednesday the 16th June for the Royal meeting. Lotus were terrific in the help they provided and the other sponsors were so generous with donations for the prize draws. We ended up with some magnificent prizes including an all-inclusive holiday to Saint Lucia, a fabulous five day trip to the Dubai World Cup and a weekend at the Prix de L'Arc de Triomphe. I'd have liked to win a few of those myself. All in all we raised about £180,000 and I achieved a first as no one had ever visited all 60 courses on consecutive days. I'd also like to thank my good friends

Roger Shelton and Colin McKenzie who were co-navigators for parts of the journey.

In 2015 The Bob Champion Research and Education Building opened in Norwich. Professor Cooper had said that Norwich was the upcoming place to be and he was right. We decided to open the new research facility within the Norwich Research Park, which is operated by the University of East Anglia in partnership with the Norfolk and Norwich University Hospital.

Our centre provides state-of-the-art laboratories for a small team of researchers to explore new treatments for diseases from prostate cancer and antibiotic resistance, to musculo-skeletal and gastrointestinal diseases. I'll be honest, it wasn't until recently that I fully understood what they're doing, as it is by its nature very technical and complicated, but I was lucky enough to spend some time listening to Colin explain what's happening.

I think the most amazing development is that the Trust is now funding research to develop a urine test that can diagnose prostate cancer and ultimately, determine whether the prostate cancer is the aggressive type. However, as to how they're doing that, I should probably get Professor Cooper to explain:

"In 2011 I found myself in a situation where I had to set up my laboratory again from scratch in Norwich. It was funding from the Bob Champion Cancer Trust and from The Grand Charity (now the Masonic Charitable Foundation) that allowed me to do this. In particular the Bob Champion Cancer Trust funded an item of equipment that cost £100,000 and would form the foundation of my work over the next few years. It was this item of equipment (a fluorescence microscope) that led to the identification of bacteria in urine that are associated with the development of prostate cancer. Without this funding this important work would not have happened."

Can you imagine simply taking a urine test to get a diagnosis and know what kind of treatment is actually required? Professor Cooper continues:

> *"The Bob Champion Cancer Trust funded two posts in my laboratory. A postdoctoral worker called Rachel Hurst, who works on the identification of bacteria in urine. This is work that will determine if bacterial infection is linked to cancer development. The second post is Dan Brewer who was funded for a time from the Bob Champion Trust money. While he was receiving this funding he discovered the DESNT poor prognosis cancer category together with myself, a PhD student called Bogdan Luca and Vincent Moulton, the head of computing.*
>
> *At one point in the project we were using 12% of UEA's computing capacity ongoing and you have to realise that is a significant amount of computer power. I should say that this is a remarkable piece of work that effectively solved the "tiger-pussycat" problem. That is distinguishing aggressive from non-aggressive prostate cancer and allowing therapy to be targeted to the men that need it, avoiding impotence in men who would be treated unnecessarily. I consider this as the most important achievement of my career and it was funded by the Bob Champion Cancer Trust."*

When someone like Professor Cooper says that the Trust's money helped him with the most important achievement of his already very distinguished career, everything we have done with the Trust is absolutely worth it and everyone who has ever donated a penny or a pound should be very proud of themselves.

He mentions Dr Rachel Hurst, who happens to be one of the nicest and most excited people I've ever met when it comes to wee! She explained to me that you can see the whole of the prostate when looking at urine samples and so it's far easier to detect abnormalities. The research lab combining Rachel's findings have now started looking at bacteria as a trigger for prostate cancer. Having examined 340 samples Dr Hurst recognised that there was a correlation between the type of bacteria present in the urinary tract and the seriousness of the prostate cancer.

When looking at prostate cancer Professor Cooper always refers to it as the 'tigers and pussycats' as there are different forms, some requiring far less aggressive treatment. Currently it hasn't been possible to determine if a patient has a more or less aggressive form and therefore they can often be given unnecessary treatments. The researchers hope that by identifying the bacteria they can help to better diagnose the form of prostate cancer and save patients receiving medication they don't need.

Initially research had followed the same route as breast cancer with researchers looking at a simple math equation for identifying subtypes of cancer, but this simply wasn't successful. However in the last year there has been a breakthrough whereby using a far more sophisticated math framework has led to the identification of an aggressive subtype. The next stage will be to start clinical trials to see how effective the results are at identifying prostate cancer early and eventually eradicating it entirely. I was astounded that bacteria could well be the cause of prostate cancer and if this is proven to be the case, then, if discovered early enough it could be prevented by antibiotics. How amazing would that be?

Treatment of prostate cancer has improved dramatically over the years, but it is this issue of who to treat, the tigers and the pussycats, that remained the critical problem. It is such a great thing that the Bob Champion Cancer Trust has helped in Professor Cooper and his team's big success.

Aside from the amazing achievements there have been a few funny incidents. Professor Cooper reminded me of the time we took Aldaniti to the centre and as horses do, he left a parcel of manure outside the building. One of the researchers was torn between selling it on eBay or putting it on his garden. We think his garden won in the end!

There was also the time when Professor Cooper and his team had been invited to a function at the Palace, to be properly recognised for their fund raising and research.

He says,

"I was so thrilled at the thought of meeting the Queen and quite nervous, but in the end she walked straight past me and went to see the horse! Very humbling, but you could see she had a genuine affection there."

In 2016 we got involved with the Shetland Pony Grand National when they nominated us as their charity for the year. You know I love these races and I try to get to as many of the qualifiers as I can. Often it's the children of jockeys that you see coming through on the ponies and it is simply great fun. The qualifiers are held throughout the year and then the National itself is at Olympia in December. It's an incredible spectacle and if you've never seen Shetlands race then I urge you to take a look on the Internet. These little horses can't half move and they are so full of spirit. The kids are fantastic and not at all fazed by the jumps or indeed the crowd which is always huge.

I often get to hook up with Derek at those events and when I asked him about them he gave me the same old story he always does:

"I walked into the ring with Bob and he pushed me forward to be introduced, he's just so quiet and unassuming. However when he was announced the crowd burst into life clapping, cheering and whistling. It's so very humbling to stand with him when that happens. Whilst the children there may not know who he is or what he's achieved, the parents do and they've never forgotten, it makes you proud to be there with him."

Yeah, yeah… Derek says things like that but on the night he'll be telling me they're cheering him!

This last year of 2017 the Shetland Pony Grand National have kindly nominated us again as their charity and we've had great fun supporting all of the children involved.

In April 2017 I had the pleasure of being invited to attend the Oakbank Easter Racing Carnival on behalf of the Australian Cancer Trust. I flew out on the Thursday evening, arrived in Adelaide on the Friday night and had drinks with those organising the event. We went to the races on the Saturday and had dinner in the evening. On the Sunday I went to a charity event where I met with the remarkable former jockey and now racing journalist, John Letts, who is amazingly funny and a really talented presenter. He's one of those people I instantly liked when I met him. Then it was back to the races on the Monday, flew out Monday night and arrived home Tuesday afternoon in time to go racing at Newmarket. Then it was onto Cheltenham on the Wednesday, staying over with Nigel and Sally before attending another Legend's Race at Cheltenham Racecourse on the Thursday, in aid of our Trust and the Hannah's Willberry Wonder Pony. It may sound glamorous but I can assure you that at times it's absolutely exhausting. However, if you ask me when I'll retire, I'll tell you I won't. The Trust is a huge part of my life. The money we raise makes a difference and that is worth any amount of jetlag or sleepless nights. If I can help just one person not go through what I did, it will be more than worth it.

Almost thirty-five years of fundraising has seen us collectively raise almost £15M. We are extremely thankful to so many individuals for raising funds, but a special thank you must be said to Simon Massen and his Committee 'Campaign Care', who over the years have held various events and raised approximately £200,000.

In summing up the charity I'll leave it to the words of one of my co-founders, Nick Embiricos, when he said, "We're not a pain in the arse sort of charity. We don't badger people for money, we always try to raise money in a nice way."

Before we leave the Trust and move onto what happened in the rest of my life after the National, it is a sad fact that a lot of people I have met over the years have passed away because of cancer. Many more, who helped raised funds and gave so generously of their time have also gone, to old age or other causes. Yet there was one individual, without whom we wouldn't have had any of it.

On the 28th March 1997, I received the devastating news that Aldaniti had passed away. He hardly appeared anymore at Trust events by then as he was twenty-seven years old and getting on. He was living his life with Nick and Valda, totally happy and not a little spoilt. He'd had a few minor heart scares the week before, but on this particular morning they let him out of his stall and he ran in the paddock, as he did every morning. Then, he simply died. Lying down on a fresh spring morning under a sky of bright white clouds with a stroke of blue peeking through, for all the world looking like the colours I had the privilege of wearing when he carried me to my greatest triumph.

Nick called me to break the news and I was so upset. I had loved that horse from the moment I first sat on him at Ascot and I had known right from the outset that he was one of the special ones. He didn't suffer and died where he was happy. I was heartbroken. He'd been a part of my life for so long and he was in a way part of me. He's buried in the paddock where he died and a part of him is and always will be, carried in my heart.

Heavy Going

In the weeks following the 1981 National, I made my way to Ascot, had a fall and shattered a few vertebrae. Technically I suppose you could call it a broken back. It wasn't the ideal way to finish off my triumphant season, but what with the book and the donations to the Royal Marsden and all the attendant publicity, some may have thought it maybe wasn't a bad thing to have an enforced rest from riding. They wouldn't be jockeys though. I found it frustrating.

Once recovered and yes, I mean recovered enough, and with only three days before the race itself, I was invited to ride in the New Zealand Grand National. Having agreed to race in a moment of madness, I then called back to find out what my racing weight would need to be. I was gutted to hear I needed to lose 10lb, so it was three grim days of saunas and not eating, although as twenty-four hours were spent travelling it wasn't as bad as it could have been. I somehow managed to lose the weight and got to New Zealand in plenty of time.

Just after I arrived in the jockey's room, a dour looking man walked in. My stomach dropped as I had a rotten feeling he was looking for me. Sure enough he called my name and came over to tell me my horse had been pulled! I couldn't believe it. I'd flown halfway around the world to be on a non-runner. Someone felt guilty enough to put me on a horse to parade around and do the celebrity bit and then it was back to the airport for a flight home. Of course the air traffic controllers had other ideas.

Over the next five days, airports across the world were going to be affected by strikes and on this occasion several back-to-back delays meant that I could either sit in airline lounges, or, a little ahead of a planned schedule, go and see my old friend Burly Cocks. It's funny as I look back on that trip, I can see it was another cross-roads in my life. Whilst I was out with Burly he offered me a really good opportunity, a decent training job and I'm sure, had I been single I would have stayed. I really think I could have had an amazing life over there, but I wasn't single anymore. In fact I was in the middle of wedding plans. I can safely say, that had I not been, I would have jumped at the opportunity. Of course you can't go back and change things, but if I could, then this would definitely be one of the reset points in my life. As it was, I came home to England and a few days after my return I was invited to ride in the newly named, 'Bob Champion Chase' which to my delight, I won. It seemed I would return to my usual life, but in reality what with the mounting publicity, the book and the overtures from film companies, that 81-82 season I was two-thirds a jockey. I also continued to struggle with my weight, had a few bad falls and added to all of that, was looking forward to becoming a settled man with a girl called Jo.

I first met Jo Beswick in 1976 and we dated casually. It was rather an off and on arrangement that suited both of us. She had been an amateur jockey who always rode well, was fun to be around and we shared similar interests. She had worked in America for a while and had been there towards the end of my cancer treatments and through the start of my recovery. Eventually, as 1980 progressed into 1981, we began to spend more time together and I realised that my feelings for her were deeper than anything I had felt before. Whilst I might have been known as a ladies man, I was in no doubt that she was the one.

Being shy, it took all my courage to make the proposal and I was chuffed when she said yes. We spent a year together before we were to get married and it was a really good time. It's strange how your mind and memories work. Even though we would go on to get divorced and our relationship would sour and become toxic, she was with me when I won the National and so, in that memory, on that day in Aintree, she is there smiling, in happier times.

We got married on the 12th October 1981 and, in hindsight, our relationship was placed under pressure from day one. Literally. With so much happening in my life, the marriage and indeed the actual wedding itself was at the centre of a hectic whirlpool of attention and celebrity. We never really had a chance to spend time and learn about each other as most newlyweds do.

Going into the marriage I was of course convinced this was it for life. Not everyone it seemed shared my opinion, although only one person voiced it out loud. I went to see Val Ridgeway the morning of the wedding as I'd been racing the day before and had been badly bruised. Val was helping to get me back on my feet like she always did.

As I was leaving she said, "You're doing the wrong thing this afternoon, you know?"

Perhaps had more people spoken up they could have saved me from what turned out to be not such a happily ever after.

When I say the pressure started on day one, I mean it. The spotlight of publicity fell on us as we walked out of the church. Not that I knew about it, but it had all been arranged for This Is Your Life to be filmed on that very afternoon.

Sally and Nigel, my friends who had made me the gift of the horseshoe at Aintree, were with me on the morning of the wedding and they walked to church with me. I remember asking them to walk either side of me as they were both taller than me and I hoped that they would screen me from the waiting press. Of course I didn't know at the time, but they were fully aware that Eamonn Andrews was waiting to pounce on me the moment the service was over and no amount of screening would work.

It's no longer on TV, but 'This is Your Life' was a huge deal back then. It was a show, for those who may never have seen it, which surprised a well-known person and told their life story through the memories of others. From parents to long lost friends to those that you might not have even realised you'd had an influence on. Looking back, it was a bit cheesy, but at the time it was a really nice thing to have happen and was a celebration of family and friends. You can find various episodes, mine included I suppose, if you look hard enough on YouTube. The surprise 'pouncing' on the subject person was key and there was a great deal of effort put into not letting the unsuspecting 'star' know they were to feature. They did it really well with me, I honestly had no idea. My only inkling had been that the marquee set up for the reception seemed a lot bigger than I had remembered us planning, but I figured Jo had decided to invite a few more friends and that was fine by me.

Although it was a lovely honour, I can't help but think that to have a TV show filmed on your wedding day was a bit weird. I was surprised, not only by being confronted by 'the big red book' but also I didn't think many women would really want the focus of the day to be on the groom, but Jo had gone along with the whole thing and helped arrange it. I'm really pleased she did. It was a great day and to be fair, the filming didn't take too long. The production company and all the crew knew what they were about and it flowed very smoothly. Obviously there were some very old friends and family in attendance and I was just relieved that I knew everyone that turned up. I was especially humbled when Burly Cocks and his wife, Babs, were brought in. They had come all the way from the States and said some really nice and heart-warming things about me. Not to be outdone, Ian Watkinson had travelled from Australia and probably had less nice things to say, but he had to behave for the cameras! I was very touched. I do remember looking across at Mary when she came in and whispering, "I'm not giving you a hug."

She shoved me and said, "I wasn't giving you one anyway, we're not the hugging type."

One of the other bonuses of the filming was that I didn't have to do all the standing in line to greet wedding guests! Funny that isn't it? I know some that would love all that, but I have to agree with Mary, I'm not the hugging type and standing in a line with people shaking your hand and most of them wanting a hug wasn't for me. Aside from the occasional peck on the cheek I'm not one for great shows of affection.

Jo and I didn't get to go on a honeymoon as I only had a few days off for the wedding. In fact I'd ridden two winners two days before it and the day after it I was straight back to being a jockey. As I've mentioned, I was two-thirds focussed. I enjoyed a few successes but once again, the target for me was an April return to Aintree. I thought it would be my grand finale. I was wrong of course. The omens were there for me to see, but I did my best to steadfastly ignore them.

In February 1982, Aldaniti, under the guidance of Ron Barry as I was injured, ran in his first outing for the season at Newbury. Historically the horse always ran well, if not won his first start, but this year he laboured and came in a disappointing fourth. I was perturbed, but not too badly.

Much worse, in the weeks leading up to the big race, the jockey world received some terrible news.

John Thorne, second to me on Spartan Missile in '81 and an absolute gentleman, was rushed to hospital on the 6th March after a fall in a Bicester point-to-point. He died the following day from his injuries. At fifty-four, he had so nearly become the oldest man ever to win at Aintree. How ironic then was the result of the 1982 race.

Immensely saddened by this tragedy, a couple of weeks later I nevertheless went to Cheltenham for the Festival and rode one of Josh's horses, called Spider's Well. I'd ridden him first in a hurdle race at Wetherby where he had duly obliged. Now we took him to the Novice Hurdle and he came second. It was a great ride and had he won it, I should have retired there and then, but of course I wouldn't have. I desperately wanted to take Aldaniti back to the National's Winner's Enclosure, yet I almost missed out on the opportunity altogether thanks to the stupidest horse I've ever sat on.

African Prince, slow-brained over hurdles, but who I had somehow managed to get to win over fences was thick. There's no other way to describe it. After my victory on him, I wasn't able to make weight next time out so Hywel Davies took the ride. I warned him not to lose his temper and to be gently persuasive for the opening section of the race as the horse would, eventually, figure it out. Hywel, understandably, got frustrated with him, gave him a whack going into the third and African Prince turned a complete double-somersault. I'd never seen anything like it.

Back at Newbury, the week before the National, I was once more reunited with the horse and coaxed him along gently for a circuit. I then felt a bit of confidence at bringing him into the race at the cross fence whereupon he did a treble-somersault, catapulted me off and I landed full on my head. Concussed isn't the word for it. I was completely gaga, but knew that if the course doctor saw the state I was in he'd red-card me for the big meeting, so I got back to the weighing room, threw my clothes on, grabbed my keys and did a very quick exit from the course. Thankfully the valets, as usual, sorted out all the rest of my kit and delivered it on to me. I stayed out of trouble for the next week and then it was back to Liverpool.

On the day after the Falkland Islands had been invaded, but long before we knew what that was to bring about, Aldaniti and I set out to win back-to-back Nationals. We'd be the first since Brian Fletcher and Red Rum in 1973 and '74. In a field of thirty-nine, we went off as joint-third-favourite. Like our run in '81, Aldaniti went off at the gallop and I tried to pull him in a bit as we crossed the Melling Road. Rather than slowing, if anything he and the rest of the field quickened. The pace was ridiculous and I honestly don't think I've seen National runners approach that first fence faster. It told. Aldaniti and I hit it at speed and, along with a quite remarkable nine other horses, fell.

I climbed up off the turf, thinking it was time to hang up my riding boots once and for all. I walked back to the stands to see the favourite, Grittar, win easily under the amateur Dick Saunders, who at the age of forty-eight became, and remains, the oldest jockey ever to win the National. I should also give my old mate Bill Smith a nod for an outstanding piece of riding at the thirteenth fence. On board Delmoss, he was almost completely carried out of the race by a riderless horse, yet he managed to control his mount, calmed him and finished fourth on the 50-1 shot.

Of course I didn't want to actually quit my riding career on a faller and I knew that I had another opportunity to go out in a more fitting manner. Where better to finish as a jockey than in God's

Own Country? So I travelled up to Wetherby in the great county of Yorkshire and on the 12th of April had a ride on Ridan Tower. I could only manage third. Not that he was ever going to finish anything but third, I still felt that I hadn't given as good a ride as I could have. I especially felt I hadn't pushed him enough over the last ditch. Weighing in at 10st 13lb, I went off to stay overnight at Howard Thompson's and hoped the next day, Tuesday the 13th April 1982, would bring me better luck.

The horse was Lumen and when I weighed out at 11st 10lbs, an amazing 11lbs heavier than I had been the previous evening, I didn't think things were looking great. I was even more confused when the clerk of the scales told me I was supposed to have blinkers. I'd ridden for Josh for nearly ten years and we'd never used blinkers. I spoke to the Guv'nor in the parade ring.

As usual, Josh was his usual straightforward, practical self. "I think he needs them, Bob."

We put them on, I got a leg up, rode Lumen round the hurdles track to victory and recorded the last winner of my career. It was time to move on and it seemed obvious to me that I would become a trainer. Mainly because I thought it was probably the only other thing I could do. After all, I knew horses and I knew racing, that was my world and the only skills I thought I had.

On my return from Wetherby I formalised my decision that my serious riding days were done. Having sold my first house I bought another one, with some adjacent land, near Swindon and set about knocking down some of the older buildings to clear space for stables. Even though I say so myself, I did a pretty neat job. It was ready for me to build a new trainer's yard.

I wanted to be hands-on so I started building the stables and creating the yard myself. I might not be the world's best handy man but I can graft and I liked to be involved. I was also still riding out to help keep fit. I guess though I'd slacked off a fair amount and the weight was starting to creep on. It's a funny thing, 'contentment'. It does have a way of putting the pounds on and for a while I was really content. I had a home, a business and a happy home life. On the surface it looked perfect.

The stables were getting established and soon Ken Hunt was the first owner to come to me with his horses. I was very fortunate that he truly believed in me from day one. He was a kind and generous man who gave me unconditional support, staying with me throughout my training career. It saddened me immensely when he died in 2016, but at least I was pleased that I'd been able to train a lot of winners for him.

In those early days, Ken was quickly joined by Frank Pullen. I'd always ridden for Frank and when I set up as a trainer he asked me to go buy a horse that I could train for him. I went up to the Doncaster sales and every single thing I saw was either too expensive or not worth looking at. I was about to call it quits for the day when this one youngster came in. There was just something about him. I was told he'd run in a flat race the previous day, so after checking his legs out, I paid £5,000 for him.

Then I gave his former trainer, Captain Ryan Price, a ring to ask his advice.

"He's very free Bob," said the Captain. "I don't think he would be likely to win a jumps race."

I sort of wished I'd rung him before I had handed over the money.

Anyway, I took the horse to Folkestone and had John Reid, the amicable Northern Irish flat jockey, in the saddle. I told John to hold him up, which was a big mistake on my part. The horse fought the whole way round and I should have let John have the freedom to just go with him. As it was he finished nowhere.

The next day, I was still livid with myself. I schooled the horse over some fences and then took him to be gelded. A few months later I ran him for the first time over hurdles but he was much too keen and ran himself out of it. I wondered if I could get him ultra-fit and decided to ride him out myself. Poor fella had to carry my heavy weight up and down hills. After a while I took him to Fontwell for another hurdles outing and with Hywel Davies riding, I gave instructions to bounce him out, be wary of him being quick at the start but that he would likely settle. He performed as expected but still wasn't in the frame, but on the next hurdles outing, at Plumpton with Richard Rowe, he won. As he did in his next three races. After a short break I ran him over fences and he won both his starts before he developed leg problems. That was Just Martin, my first ever winner as a trainer over hurdles and fences. The fact that he was Frank Pullen's horse seemed somehow to be a fitting thank you to a man who had spent all that time sitting by my hospital bedside.

From those modest beginnings, I managed to build up a fair stables and began to see some moderate success, but I was trying to do it at the wrong time. What with the publicity, all of the interest in the book, the Trust and then the movie, my focus was being dragged away from the business of horses. Looking back now it was really too much to try and achieve, especially as only two years into my training career I would be off touring the world in the middle of a PR whirlwind. I couldn't give the horses my undivided attention and even today, if I can't give something my very best then I don't like to do it. I should have seen the writing on the wall, but of course I didn't. I was too close to the wall and all I could see was that I had to keep pushing against it.

ϕ

Sometimes when I look back I realise that I had almost a lifetime's events happen in the space of three years. It was such an incredibly moving and knackering time, almost like being swept along by a strong flowing river. Every now and again a strange little, surreal current would spin me around and leave me feeling proud, or humble, or just stunned at the generosity of people. One such event was the first big award I was given.

The BBC Sports Personality of the Year is a big event in the sporting calendar of the UK. It was first presented in 1954 and was, even then, exclusively voted on by members of the British public. I think that's why it is held in such high regards by sportspeople and has grown to be such a part of the British cultural landscape. It's a true recognition from the fans of sport and without them, we wouldn't be able to do what we do.

In 1960 the BBC introduced the Sports Personality Team of the Year Award to recognise the team that achieved the most notable performance in the calendar year to date. Although changed now, back in 1981 it too was voted on by members of the public. Unlike many awards, where you know you are getting it before the evening, this one is wrapped in secrecy, so of course I knew that Aldaniti and I had been nominated, but we really had no idea if we'd win. Mind you, there was a bit of precedence for a horse winning. Back in 1970 the Canadian Nijinsky racing team won it for the outstanding exploits of that amazing thoroughbred who had become the first horse for thirty-five years to win the English flat-racing Triple Crown. But, the Vincent O'Brien trained Nijinsky was regarded by many to have been the greatest flat racehorse in Europe during the 20th century. Aldaniti and I had won the National. There was a bit of a difference in my mind. Still, I well knew by then how the 'battler' nature of our story had touched the British public, so although I really didn't expect it, I wasn't completely surprised when they called our name.

Being given the award and having the recognition of the public for what we had achieved was an incredible thing. For me, the walk to the stage was one of the most nerve-wracking experiences in my life. To the right and left and everywhere I looked, were so many famous sporting legends. I was seriously in awe. These were some of my sporting heroes and here they all were, watching me go up to collect an award.

Although I have to say, all of the special moments of that evening are eclipsed in my mind by one in particular. Whilst the award itself was a great acknowledgement of all the hard work put in by Josh and Nick and the team, as well as Aldaniti, the absolute highlight for me was meeting Muhammad Ali. He truly was 'The Greatest' and I'll never forget seeing him. He was a man I admired, a true legend and it is so sad that he has passed.

By the time of that award, the book had been released and on the back of it, I began to get requests to speak at functions. The number of these speaking arrangements began to grow as it seemed I was considered something of a motivator and an inspiration to others. I didn't see it that way, but I was happy to talk to people and tell them my story. I figured it was probably an easy thing to do, although the very first time I tried it was a near disaster and gave rise to my hate of autocues.

I'd probably recommend to any would-be speakers out there, to perhaps build up slowly towards this new venture in your life. I didn't. My first professional speaking engagement was in 1982. A motivational talk in front of 5,000 insurance sales people at Wembley Stadium; nothing like starting small eh? I recall that someone had written the speech for me and it had far too many S's in it! I was completely out of my comfort zone, nervous and struggling like a madman to keep up with an autocue that was travelling quite fast and didn't seem to be in any particular need to stop for me to get all these S's out. Oh, it wasn't good and I just about stumbled my way through it. I'm sure they must have thought I was a right idiot. A few weeks later I was to speak at the NEC in Birmingham, yeah I know, go small again Bob... but before it I was chatting to David Coleman. He'd watched me rehearse and could see me struggling with the autocue and speech problem.

He said, "Just use the bits you want Bob, you don't have to read it as it's written. Say what feels comfortable to you."

Well this was a relief, so I started off with the autocue but stopped using it and just said what was in my mind. I haven't used one since.

I don't really write a speech at all anymore. I will make a note about the event that I'm at but it's there in my heart. I talk to people about what affected me, what drove me and more importantly how you can use your achievements to help others. I have lost count of the number of after dinner engagements I've spoken at, so I figure I must be okay for them to ask me back again! I now travel around the UK on a weekly basis to attend functions, it's a chance to help others and to give back although the 1,000miles of road time most weeks can be a great source of frustration, given the state of some of our roads. Add to that the occasional tractor in front of me and I do revisit my idea of standing for parliament just to introduce some new road laws. But perhaps I shouldn't as I don't have much time for politicians in general, although I did once, memorably, receive a letter direct from the Cabinet Office.

φ

In the May of 1982, a very official envelope landed on my hall carpet. When I opened it, I stared down at one of those surreal moments I mentioned, but this one was huge. Nothing prepares you for it. Well, certainly not me. The letter said, "Her Majesty the Queen may be graciously pleased to approve that you be appointed a Member of the Most Excellent Order of the British Empire (MBE) in the Queen's Birthday Honours List". Apparently the Prime Minister wanted to know if it would be 'agreeable' to me. I thought, who would turn it down, you know? It was an amazing thing to be offered, so yes, of course I would accept it.

I'd been very fortunate to meet the Queen on a number of occasions before this and on each she'd always taken the time to stop and speak, particularly if I had Aldaniti with me. As with most of the Royal Family, Her Majesty is extremely fond of horses and racing and was always delighted to see him, but I had never expected to be honoured by her.

I couldn't tell anyone about the upcoming award and then finally it was announced in the London Gazette on the 12th June. After that, all I had to do was wait for my investiture date to be confirmed. Although the Birthday Honours and New Year Honours are always announced at the same time each year, the actual awarding of the medals are spaced out over months. I can't actually remember an awful lot about the build up to it, but I know I went out and hired a morning suit. I figured that I could have bought one but I didn't really think I'd get that much wear out of it. After all, how often would I need to be dressed up all posh? Mum and Jo were invited and went to town of course. Mum was working for a top class dress designer back then, doing alterations, so I know she looked absolutely fantastic.

Mum was my fan club and if I could have only taken one person with me that day it would have been her. She was a mixture of nerves and happiness and pride in me. It was a wonderful thing for a son to witness. Obviously impressed with the pomp and splendour of it all, I can recall her being somewhat put out that the toilets in Buckingham Palace weren't that special. She did reckon that the ones for the Royal Family were probably far better! We arrived and were given champagne and ushered into a special waiting room where other award recipients were also waiting. A Court official tells you what you need to do when you are receiving your award and then we were left alone. Mum, Jo and I chatted nervously with a few people and my most prevalent memory is that it felt quite scary, even though you knew it was a good thing. Then we were all asked to line up and one by one, in order, we were called forward. It's all very precise. You move forward a bit more and then you enter the main investiture hall. It's huge, with massively high ceilings and all decked out in red velvet and lots of gold. Exactly what you would expect really. I stood in front of a military officer until they called, "Civil Division, Robert Champion for services to racing" and then I went up to be presented to the Queen. I approached and bowed and she pinned the medal on me and then asked me a couple of questions. As is my way, I'm sure I asked her about a horse she'd had running the previous day! Then she shook my hand and I stepped back and bowed again and then that was that. It was over so quickly once presented with the medal. It could be compared to a production line as it was so efficiently done. We went off for lunch and by teatime I was back in the yard helping to muckout stables! I know it sounds a bit of an anti-climax but that's really what happened. I keep my medal in the bedside cabinet. My best memory of the whole day and the one that always makes me smile; my Mum was so thrilled.

φ

During all of this time I still felt very much a failure as a man, due to believing I would never be able to have children. I'd had sperm tests done even before the chemo and they'd come back negative, so I felt that there was simply no chance. Jo had assured me this wasn't an issue for her and we looked forward to the future together. Yet still that inability to have kids was sitting heavy on me. Like most things, you never know what's really important to you until you lose it. I had seemingly lost it, so you can imagine how delighted I was when, in 1983, we found she was pregnant. My baby seemed like a miracle and I couldn't believe my luck. The doctors were astounded, especially as it was so soon after the treatment, only twenty months. To be given a gift like this was unbelievable. I remember so clearly her telling me. It was one of the two proudest and happiest days in my life. The doctors were keen for me to talk about it as they felt that it gave real hope for others in my situation. Young men who would feel as I did, that having cancer would rob them of their chance at a family, might now see that there was hope.

Hope. It's such a massively important thing for all cancer sufferers and the lifebelt that they can cling on to.

The pregnancy went as well as these things can and Jo delivered a bouncing baby boy. A son, Michael. Would he become a jockey like me? After all he was the ninth generation of huntsmen bloodline.

However, after the initial excitement and thrill, I was distraught when I discovered that Michael had a heart problem and would need surgery at only six weeks old. It's something that you can't comprehend. I was terrified that we would lose him. At the time and even now if I am honest, a part of me believes that his condition was related to my cancer treatment and although this was discounted by all my doctors, I still blamed myself.

Mary recalls it was one of the first times she saw me cry. As I have said we're a tough breed but there are some events that hit you so hard that you can't accept they're happening and this was one. I tried to do things my way, focussed on the things that I could control, training and racing, but deep down there were no thoughts other than the fear that my son would die.

We were again blessed and Michael came through the surgery well. Babies and children in general are resilient and no matter how fragile they appear, they are born with an inner strength to survive. As he grew he was a happy little boy and I was really pleased to see, that like me he loved to be around the horses and the yard. We had a bond and whilst I'm not one for showing my feelings, he was my son and I loved him.

As the months progressed I was constantly touring, promoting first the book and then the movie. I was on 103 flights that year, as well as starting the Trust and trying to build my reputation as a trainer. This all took its toll and I know looking back mistakes were made by both Jo and myself, particularly as we were still learning about each other. Although I'd known Jo for some time we hadn't really spent a lot of time in each other's exclusive company.

I was still concentrating on my training career and by now had built up a string of 40 horses at the yard in Wiltshire, but really, they were mostly low-end crap, which didn't help with finances or my reputation as a trainer. There were one or two exceptions and I did train five horses for the Queen Mother, all of which placed, but sadly no winners. Her Majesty would often come for breakfast and I was able to pull her leg and make her laugh. I've said before but it's worth repeating, she was truly a lovely person and very genuine, especially when it came to her horses. I remember her with a special fondness, she was a majestic lady in every sense of the word and a kind soul.

I know that if I was reading this and it said, 'had breakfast with the Queen Mother' I'd think I was thriving, but I wasn't. Far from it. I hadn't been able to get a mortgage on the property due to the cancer, so I had taken out a loan to do the work I wanted to. It was okay, but I needed more and they would only lend it to me at ridiculous rates. I know at one point it was at a premium rate of twenty percent. There was no way I could afford that and eventually I had to sell up the yard. It was a real kick in the proverbials that I couldn't get help and the damned cancer seemed to be haunting me. Somehow it was mocking me that despite having beat it, it was always going to be a part of me. A shadow on my life, which I might never be free of.

Image Set C:

1. At a charity event in Sandringham with HRH Prince Charles and Simon Massen
2. Outside the Bob Champion Research and Education building, Norwich with Professor Colin Cooper
3. Mum and Dad at the premiere of Champions, 1984
4. The Shetland Pony Grand Nationals
5. With Michael
6. Arriving back from the gallops on Mr Felix
7. Proud of Mary, the Mayor of Royal Wootton Bassett
8. With Janette at Ben and Henri's wedding
9. Proud day giving Henri away
10. Janette and her daughters, Sam and Vicki
11. At a photo signing with the legend, Lester Piggott
12. In Dunkirk with Derek
13. Spending time with Howard
14. Having a laugh on the job!
15. Having a coffee with Ian Watkinson and Derek
16. On a polo horse in India
17. The complete line-up for the Real Marigold Hotel, 2017
18. With Stephanie Beacham, Susan George and the 'King' of India, for the Real Marigold Hotel, 2017
19. At the hotel in India with Susan George, Stephanie Beacham and Selena Scott
20. The lads in India!
21. My fetching headdress

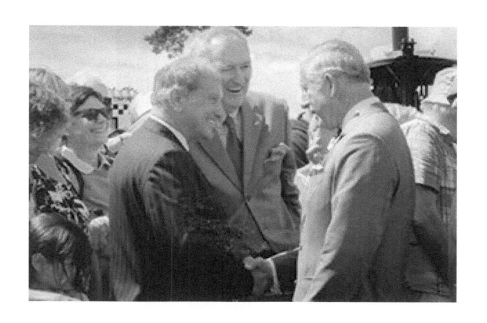

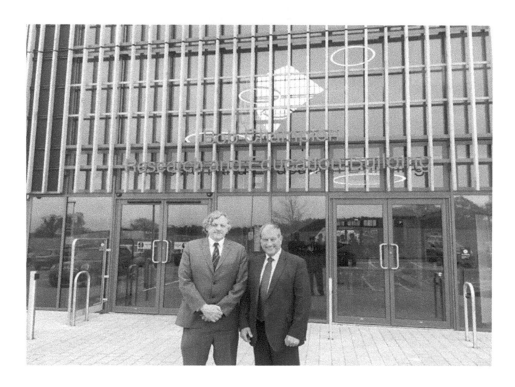

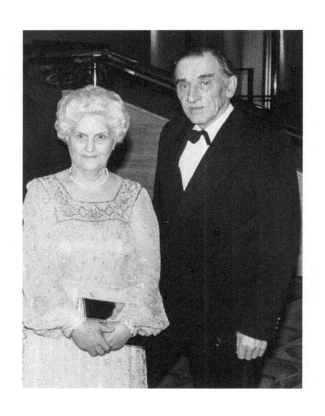

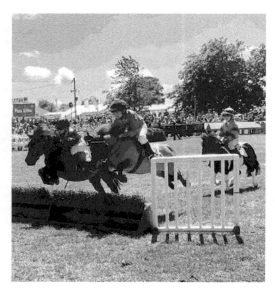

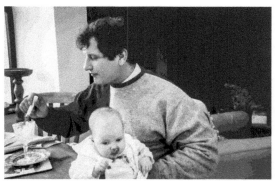

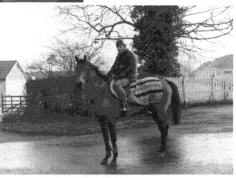

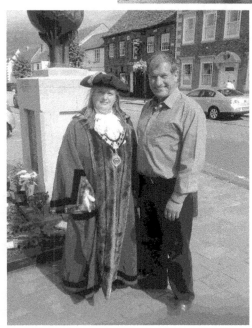

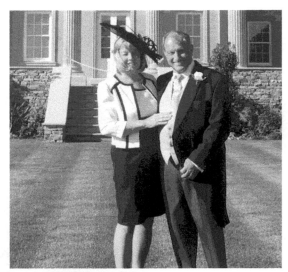

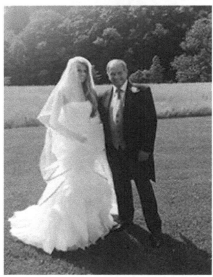

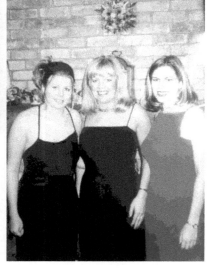

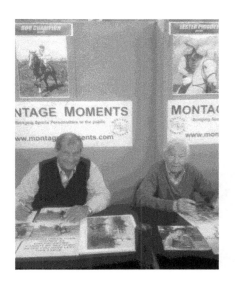

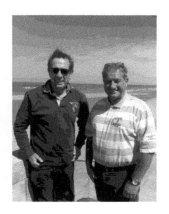

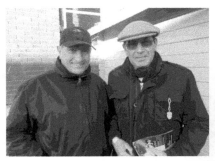

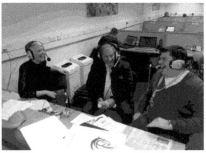

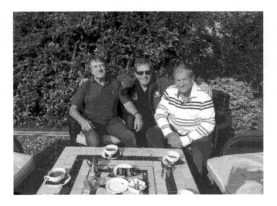

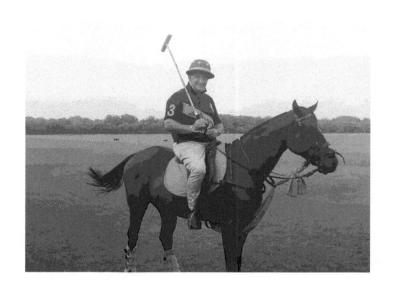

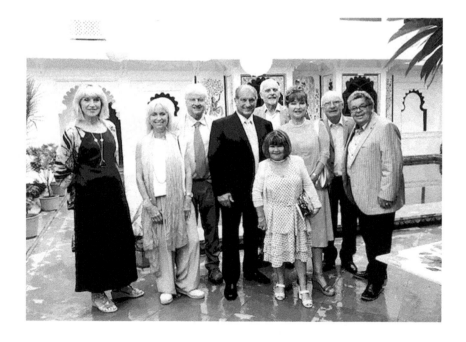

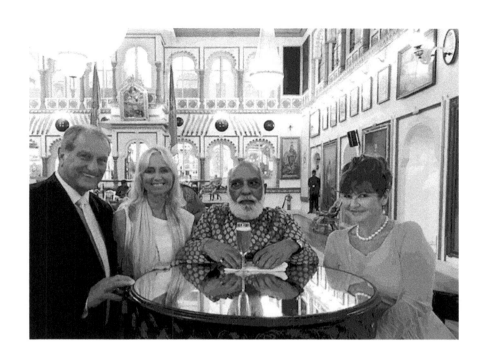

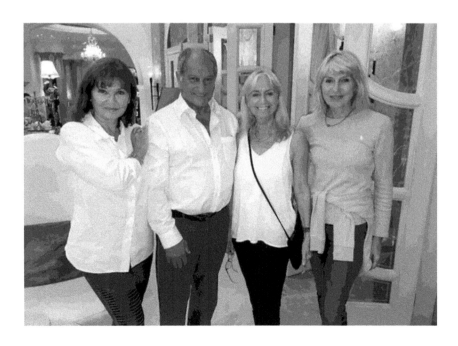

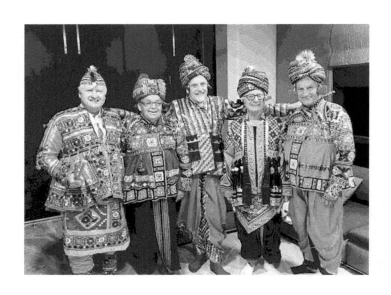

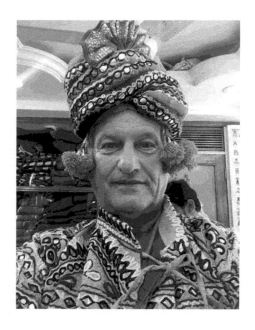

The stupid thing was that I had so much equity in the property and in my opinion the bank was very short-sighted. I don't hold many grudges in life, but I'll never forgive them for costing me my home and my business. So self-important and utterly stupid, is it any wonder it was big banks that drove the country into such a financial disaster years later.

When you don't want to leave a place, it's remarkable how quickly it will sell. I rented a smaller yard in Bury St Edmonds, Suffolk and started to build up the stables again. I was lucky that I had a great team around me that were able to manage things whilst I was still away with the publicity machine. It was really hard going but I'm nothing if not a thick-skinned and stubborn Yorkshire man and of course I couldn't see that I was trying to do too much all at once.

As you've read, I got the call while I was in Australia that the bank was showing up an irregularity. Given that I thought everything was fine, you can possibly understand my devastation to come home to find that Jo had left, taking Michael with her. What followed was a very difficult time both emotionally and financially and not something I'd ever imagined I'd go through.

I do, of course, have regrets. Mostly losing touch with Michael. I did try, but maybe I didn't try hard enough, maybe there were other things I could have done, but at the time, I needed to try to re-establish my life and my career, so I worked. I worked all the hours I could. Initially I tried to keep the contact with Michael as regular as possible and would have him at weekends when I could, but one night, a few hours after dropping him off, I fell asleep at the wheel and wrote my car off by hitting a roundabout. Luckily there was no one else involved but it jolted me. I thought, to keep seeing Michael but to keep him safe, I could have my secretary, Jane pick him up and drop him off. That idea came to an end abruptly the following week when she was involved in an accident on a motorway and wrote my second car off. It wasn't her fault and thankfully Michael hadn't been with her at the time, but I realised that the mileages involved were simply dangerous. Slowly, the weekends became fewer and then my access was made more difficult. It did, like most of these episodes, end up in court. That's never going to be for the best. I can understand divorcing couples falling out bitterly, but I have never understood what drives people to makes the kids play a central role.

I briefly managed to keep seeing Michael and when I remarried a few years later, he would come and stay with us. Several years later, a private comment that I made in anger was to destroy my relationship with my son.

When you have an element of celebrity in your life, there will always be someone willing to write a story. Occasionally, the more salacious the better. I made an angry outburst and it was shared with a member of the media. The press attention was aimed at me and intended to shame me, yet really all it did was hurt Michael. We became estranged and I haven't seen my son since my daughter Henri's wedding in 2015. He has his own family now, doesn't want contact and I fully respect that.

Without a wife or child, I fell back on the mainstay of my life, horse racing and began to get a few winners here and there. About this time, I had one of my favourite owners, Major Eldred Wilson come on board. His only requirement of me was that his horses ran in the Grand Military Gold and Royal Artillery Gold Cup. Both of those races are restricted to currently serving military amateur riders and ownership is also limited to serving or ex-serving members of the armed forces. The former Major certainly qualified as an owner as did a certain Colonel-in-Chief to many a Regiment, Her Majesty, Queen Elizabeth, The Queen Mother.

I ran Prydel in the Grand Military Gold Cup and although he wasn't a great jumper he got round well that day and had a photo finish with Special Cargo, one of the best National Hunt horses the Queen Mother ever owned. The Major was very familiar with the Royal Family as his farm was owned by the Crown and he often had their horses throughout the summer.

As we waited for the photo finish he said to Her Majesty, "Well Ma'am, I hope that the photograph goes your way."

I said, "Well Ma'am, I hope it goes my way!" She laughed and it went her way. In fact Special Cargo lifted that cup three times in a row and also won the Whitbread Gold Cup in what was described by Fred Winter as the greatest race he'd ever seen and he'd seen a fair few.

Major Wilson also sponsored a race at Fakenham that we entered. I'm pleased to say that every year we had a winner so he was always happy.

I also went over to Ireland and bought Turn Blue very cheaply for about £5,000. I would ride him out and the day before a race at Doncaster I took him out to Warren Hill. Henry Cecil was there and I asked if he minded me tracking his horses. Of course being the gentleman he was he said no problem and off I went. Afterwards he said, "If it jumps, it won't get beat."

I don't know what he'd seen to make him say that but he wasn't wrong. I think for me this was the type of boost I needed. With Jo and Michael gone, I was on my own and feeling quite down at the time. When you're like that you can be very hard on yourself. Having invested the time and effort in Turn Blue, it was really rewarding to see that it paid off. It was also nice to see I hadn't lost my 'eye' and that a genius like Henry agreed with me.

Shortly after, I went back to the States to see another genius, Burly Cocks, be inducted into the National Museum of Racing and Hall of Fame in Saratoga. There was no way I was going to miss that as he'd done so much for me. He was such a fantastic man and thoroughly deserved that honour.

Sometimes I wonder if during life I have ever expressed properly the debt I owed to some people. Burly was certainly one, without whom, I would never have made it back into racing. His kindness, support and loyalty were so important to my return. When he died in 1986 I was gutted. He was 82 by then but it was still sad to lose him. He'd believed in me when many hadn't and I considered him one of the mentors in my life, as of course was my Father.

My Dad often came to the yard to help out. He was old school when it came to training horses and boy did he know his stuff. His advice was often hard but invaluable and some of his ideas would today probably be seen as bordering on barbaric, but they worked. I recall when younger we had a pony that wouldn't stop rearing up.

Dad told me to get a small bottle and to fill it with blood from the knackers yard, which I did. The next time the horse reared I was to pour the blood over the horse's head and into its face. He said that the horse would think the blood was his and that the rearing up had caused it. He was absolutely right. Not only did the horse never rear again, it became quite a sound jumper. Dad also had views on feed. I was going through a bit of a lean period with winners when he stopped by one day and I was moaning to him. He looked in the feed bins and told me what I was doing wrong.

"Go back to the old ways of feeding," he advised and so I changed back to a mixture of oats with a bit of bran and bran mash twice a week. You could never fault his advice and once I changed the feed I began to get the results I wanted. Our relationship changed over the years and our initial testosterone bashing days had long since ended. I know he was very proud of all my achievements even though he might not have said as much. If I had questions about the horses or indeed the yard he would usually know the answers and I trusted his judgement. It's one of life's good things that my father stayed around long enough for his son and him to become trusted friends. I think of him often, since he passed away on 10th July 1987. It was one of those deaths that you think was so tragically sudden yet mercifully quick. Of course, the swiftness amplified the shock and the hurt.

He had lung cancer and died within a few short weeks of being diagnosed. A heavy smoker all his life it wasn't all that surprising a condition, but the speed with which it went through him was difficult to comprehend. His heavy smoking is the reason I never did. I would hear him coughing every morning and think, 'that's not for me.' I did try a cigarette once but I didn't like the taste so added to the coughing, I was truly put off. An awful lot of my contemporary jockeys used to smoke as it helped them to keep the weight down, but it wasn't for me.

Dad had complained of back ache at first and then he just began to feel unwell. Then he was gone. It was a blow to everyone, but Mum was devastated. They had been together so many years and his loss was hard on her. For me, I'd lost a mentor and a man I would always admire.

φ

I was slowly getting the yard together but was still being pulled this way and that for publicity. However, given how the Trust was fairing, which you'll have read about earlier, I had to keep up a profile, so when invites came from television shows I would often take them up. I still get invites nowadays actually, but back then it was like a blizzard of requests. I did a lot but the more memorable were Bullseye in 1984, '3-2-1' in 1987 and the Krypton Factor in 1989. That last one was a bit strange as the celebrities weren't allowed to do every round. In the end the lovely Sally Jones won and the whole experience of it and all the others was really good fun. I was even asked to do Ready-Steady-Cook, although I'm pretty sure there was a fix put in to that one, as my food looked so much tastier than Brian Turner's did and he won! It did, honestly.

Also about then I began to get calls inviting me to speak, or judge at horse shows and that's how I met my second wife, Dee in 1987.

We arranged to meet for a drink one evening to discuss a charity event and started dating from there. Dee was a butcher's daughter who came from money and was now accustomed to being around horses. Spending time with her and her two young daughters it was nice to be part of family life again and often back then, Michael would come and stay with us. I hoped that Dee would help mend bridges with Jo and Michael, but ultimately this was to backfire spectacularly.

Dee and I built that second yard together and initially we had a great marriage. She was a nice person and a really good judge of horses. Moving into the early nineties, we consistently had fifteen horses in training and we continued getting some winners, although never really enough to make the break through into the top training ranks. It also didn't help when I was quoted as saying I needed to withdraw from fundraising to spend more time on my job as a trainer. I did have a reputation as a fundraiser and owners didn't have the belief that I was dedicated enough to training and so were reluctant to bring their horses to me. To be fair I was putting in a lot of hours driving all over the country and so they weren't necessarily wrong. I did cut back on some of the charity events but it wasn't for long and I knew deep down that it was the Trust that held my true passion. However, I continued to run both lives in parallel and I think my favourite winner from that second yard came in 1993, with Pat's Minstrel over in Ireland. He won the Southampton Goodwill Handicap Chase at the Listowel Festival in County Kerry, and it really meant a lot to me. Not because of the race, or my share of the £3,943 prize money, but because of its owner, Ken Hunt.

Ken loved the horse but following two back to back successes in the March, the handicapper had really gone after Pat's Minstrel and given the weight he was to carry, there was no way we would be getting another win on him in the UK. I took him off the track for the remainder of the season and then in the September, after a 195 day layoff, I got him ready for the Listowel Festival. It's a big event as the Irish do love their festivals and Pat's Minstrel, under the guidance of a young and simply brilliant Adrian Maguire, got up to win by a short head from the slightly ironically named, Winning Charlie. Ken had had a nice little wager on him and Adrian was delighted as he'd never won a race at Listowel before, so it truly was a great day all round. I think that winner meant the most to me you know. I do recall we stopped off on the way home for dinner at a lovely hotel near Limerick, overlooking a lake. We pulled up with a horsebox and I'll never forget the doorman's face as he looked down on us, but we were in fine form and simply didn't care.

Pat's Minstrel would also be the last winner I ever trained, when he ran for me in the Jewson Handicap Chase at Fakenham in March of 1997.

But I'm getting ahead of myself, for there was something much more important that happened years before Listowel and way before Fakenham and that was having my second miracle, Henrietta, my beautiful daughter.

Again this felt like another gift, perhaps even another chance. Henri's birth on 12th October 1988 helped to mend fences with Jo and she would allow Michael to come and stay. Both of Dee's girls, Ali and Tilly, from her first marriage loved Michael and he was very much part of the family. Of course it wasn't all smooth sailing but having Henri cemented things for me. I loved being with all of the girls, they each had a very different and distinctive personality, but it was family life that I loved. I know I can look back and realise that I wasn't the warm fuzzy parent that some may love, but I was there for them and of course I was keen to help them ride and to show jump.

Unfortunately though, after a few years, I realised that the marriage wasn't working. I stayed as long as I could, trying to make the best of it, but the cracks became too large to patch. Deep down I knew that we couldn't continue as we were.

Dee and I eventually fell out irreconcilably over the running operations of the yard and I spent a long time away from home to avoid arguments. It was easier. As we had finances tied in together and I truly loved Ali, Tilly and Henrietta equally, walking away was never going to be an easy option. I always considered all of them to be my daughters, although both Ali and Tilly still saw their father.

Again I look back and think that perhaps my commitment to this marriage, like my first, wasn't completely focussed. I was probably doing too much, building the yard, PR for the Trust, attending charity functions and with all of that I didn't leave a great deal of time for family life. As usual, there was blame to be had on all sides, but I can only regret my own efforts, or lack of them. I finally realised that staying within the marriage for the sake of the kids wasn't the right thing to do either.

If I thought my break up with Jo had been bad, this was to be far, far worse. It seemed as though the time Jo and Dee had spent together had formed a bond and when the marriage broke down they joined forces. That old adage, 'Hell hath no fury like a woman scorned' needs updated to add in how furious two of them can become when united in their efforts.

I understand that I wasn't unique. I am fully aware that divorce for anyone is never easy and in my opinion, anyone that says they have had an amicable divorce is hugely lucky. For those happy souls that have never had to go through one, then thankfully they may never know what bitterness and hurt can be generated.

I know that in most divorces and relationship breakdowns there are usually three sides to the story; my truth, her truth and 'the' truth, but with the added mix of celebrity you get a fourth, the media's truth. There were, over the next few years, some horrendous stories appearing in the papers and I know that friends and family of mine encouraged me to 'get my side out' but I couldn't. I suppose some people think that as I haven't challenged the allegations against me, then there must be some fire with the smoke, but it is simply that I am firmly of the belief it's not the honourable thing to do. I am always surprised when people choose to air their dirty laundry in public. Of course it's down to the individual, but it was never going to be something I could do. The idea of a 'no holds barred' public airing of personal issues in the press was completely against what I thought was right, so I chose to keep my own counsel. More importantly, regardless of how I felt about Dee or Jo, they were the mothers of my children and I never wished to say anything that could cause my children to be upset.

My approach to it didn't lessen how hurt I felt at the things being said about me. I was accused of being a gold digger, despite never taking a penny from Dee or anything I hadn't earned and in fact I came out of a marriage with nothing yet again. From then until now I have kept my peace on this and never said anything. Basically, as I sit here now, I see no point and certainly no honour in doing so in the pages of this book. I don't need to voice my anger and besides, too many years and too much water has passed under the bridge.

I will say that the press printed what they knew would sell and boy did they print. I can't blame them for being business minded, but I know my little sister did and does. Wow did she get angry in defending her big brother. She was particularly livid at the Daily Mail and in fact wrote a letter to the editor telling them what she thought! Not one to mince words is our Mary!

Those closest to me knew the truth and stood by me. For that they have my heartfelt thanks. It's a really difficult place when you don't know which friend could turn on you and some days I dreaded opening the newspapers. You learn who the friends and acquaintances and fly-by-nights are in times like those. I know my friends and each one stood by my side.

As with the divorce from Jo, I regret one thing about the split with Dee. Just as I struggled to keep my relationship with Michael, so I lost years with Henri, Ali and Tilly too, but the universe turns and I am delighted to say that I am incredibly lucky to have them back in my life now. With everything I have done, giving life to my two kids and, despite difficult situations, being part of my step-children's lives, has been a true privilege and I have always tried to do my best by them.

ф

"I have tremendous respect for Bob and all that he has done for charity. Growing up I was ten and a half months older than Ali and I think that made a great deal of difference to my relationship with Bob in comparison to hers. At times I was awful to him, but looking back I was acting as many children do with a new step-parent.

Bob always treated us as his daughters and was the best teacher ever with our ponies. He would come and watch us and never reacted if we made a mistake in the ring. He always taught us to get up and get back on if we fell. He had the best hands and taught us all to ride without reins.

Bob arranged for me to have work experience with ex-jockey and now sculptor Philip Blacker and I was with him for nine years before I went to study art in Italy. I was also pleased to design one of the Christmas cards for the Trust. Recently Bob told me I needed a kick up the bum to start drawing again as I am, 'so talented' which I accept is his way of offering support! We've only recently been back in touch but I'm pleased that we are."
Tilly Taylor-Levey

Tilly has always been incredibly talented and so I am of course delighted to see her using it. I agree she was a madam at times but it was understandable!

Growing up Bob and I were joined at the hip. I wanted to go everywhere with him. I would watch National Velvet and thought of myself as Elizabeth Taylor. Being around Bob and the horses were my favourite times. Bob would pop his head in on me in the morning and if I was awake he'd give me twenty minutes to get ready and by the time I got downstairs my pony would be saddled. I would go on the gallops and then I'd dash off to get fresh bread for the lads for breakfast. It would be quite nibbled by the time I got back as I could never resist taking a bite.

He was very competitive on our behalf, especially when we were showing and he'd walk the course with us beforehand. He had a knack of explaining the course to us in a language that we understood, and always kept us calm.

He was always stubborn though and hated to be beaten, whether it was a pony that wouldn't go through water or something as silly as roller skating, some things didn't go his way! I remember Bob falling over on skates and that was it, we all had to go home!

One of my favourite memories was in taking Pat's Minstrel to Ireland. I loved that horse and being able to travel on the ferry with the jockeys and trying my first ever sip of Guinness will always stay with me. As will begging Bob to let me jump on him. I was only seven and Pat's Minstrel was a full thoroughbred racehorse. Bob put out a cavaletti in the sand which was small enough for him to walk over, the first time he lurched slightly and I tumbled off. I was more embarrassed than hurt and was straight back on, this time Bob held my leg and we went over. The horse hadn't really 'jumped', but to me it felt incredible. I remember shouting that I'd jumped Pat's Minstrel in the yard! This was Bob, he would encourage you to follow your dreams.

I have recently started having jumping lessons with him and just like when I was little there was no practice, it was straight in. He has confidence in you which makes you feel you can just do it. He is a very good teacher. I'm involved in jumping ex-racehorses and I know that he loves being involved.

One thing I will say is that he simply cannot concentrate on more than one thing at a time, he's never without his phone and is often distracted!
Ali Stearn

Ali and I shared so many hours together through the horses. At times she was very much a mini-me and I was always proud of her grit and determination. I love the fact that she's involved in working with ex-racehorses now, as this is such a valuable thing for them to have a new lease of life.

One of my proudest moments was giving Henri away when she married Ben in 2015. In fact Ben came to ask me for Henri's hand and as he's a Yorkshire man too I had no problem with saying yes. I was involved with all the preparations and the wedding itself went fantastically well. There wasn't a thing that could have dampened the pleasure of that day.

Henri looked truly stunning and there wasn't a nerve in sight with her. I had my speech ready and phone in hand so all was good. Of course there were tense moments as there is no love lost between Dee and myself, but Ben's parents were very friendly. The reception was held at their home and it was a stunning location, the perfect setting. I could see just how happy Henri and Ben were and this was more than enough for me.

"My Dad and I have always been close and we speak on a daily basis. We don't see each other as often as we'd like as we live so far apart and both have busy lives.

I married on 4th July 2015 in Bolton by Bowland and Dad was by my side.

Having him give me away was always in my plan, in fact Ben went to see Dad to ask for my hand. I know they get on really well, probably because Ben is a Yorkshire man too!

On the day, Dad helped to keep me calm and was so relaxed he was checking his emails on the phone. I'm a relaxed person like him and walking down the aisle he told me to slow down. The ceremony itself was fun as my vicar was quite the comedian, Dad and I could hardly keep a straight face. If you look back at our photos you can see that we're all laughing. His speech was lovely and I know that the day was as special to him as it was to me.

Dad has run charity events at our restaurant and hearing him talk to those suffering from cancer sums up the person that he is. He is so kind to those who are ill and he gives them hope as well as his time. I still don't know how he manages to do everything that he does."

Henri Bannister

I'd forgotten about the vicar until Henri reminded me. The man should have been a stand-up comedian, he was so funny!

Hearing what the girls have to say, reminds me how lucky I am and how truly blessed they make me feel.

So, in 1996, after leaving the marital home, I found myself starting from scratch all over again. I rented a small bungalow in Newmarket and spent a considerable time fighting with solicitors. As you can probably guess, the only winner was always going to be the solicitor's pocket and in my case this was definitely true.

When I look back I wish I could give my younger self some advice. I'd tell me not to bother with the solicitors. I'd try to convince myself to have a rationale conversation with my ex-wives instead of how it went. It might have improved things and in the long run it could have avoided a lot of mud-slinging and hurt.

A racing yard came up for sale in Newmarket, and with a large mortgage and an additional loan from owner and good friend Ken Hunt, for which I will always be grateful, my then new partner, Janette and I were able to buy it. We managed to pay Ken back within twelve months and began to rebuild the training business.

I should take this moment to introduce Janette properly. I knew her whilst I was with Dee, but we remained strictly friends until my marriage broke down. Dee went so far as to have me followed by a private investigator and a lot of nonsense was once again shipped off to the press. I remember walking past a newsagents and seeing a headline that read something like: 'Love Cheat Exposed' and thought, 'What a poor sod that must be,' only to realise they were talking about me! Many will say other things, but I know the truth. My truth. I was an unhappy man in an unhappy situation and Janette was there for me then and has been ever since. I owe her so much.

I will admit to being instantly attracted to Janette, she had a quiet reserve about her that my previous wives never had, a certain poise. She was incredibly kind and certainly knew how to dress as she always turned heads. I was particularly fond of her in her white jeans! I also noticed that her ponies were always immaculately turned out and whilst this may sound a little odd, I've always found that the way a person looks after their animals tells you a lot about them. Janette is quite a private person, but thoroughly enjoys attending events whenever she can. She is very confident and self-assured and I can honestly say that she is my rock. I know it is a glib statement and one trotted out so many times as to be a cliché, but it is an absolute truth for me. We have been through so much together and without her I would not be here, literally! We've had many TV shows filmed in our home, including 'Through the Key Hole', and she's graciously stayed behind the camera, happily leaving me to make a fool of myself! Despite many accusations levelled against her, she has retained her quiet dignity, something I have always loved about her.

I also loved Janette's daughters coming to stay at the stables. Sam and Vicki were very good show riders and Vicki loved riding out the racehorses. I would never tell her, but I used to put her on some of the trickier ones and she had such a way about her that they would ride as sweet as a nut for her. Some people simply have the nature that calms even the most temperamental of horses.

Sam is now married to Ed and they have two lovely children Thomas, 12 and Emily, 10 and I'm over the moon to be granddad to them. Thomas is a very kind young man and a real problem solver. Emily, the more sportier of the two, now plays cricket for

Essex and I have high hopes that maybe she'll play for England one day.

Back at the point of buying the Newmarket yard, I was riding out and taking on horses that had problems. As a trainer, not only do you prepare the horses for the season, setting them for the races you think are the most suitable, but you can be asked to help an owner pick a horse. It's not easy and although I loved training horses, I hated the rest that went with the job. Yet again, I have to be honest, I don't suppose I was the best person to deal with the owners. They've invested their money in a horse and have a desire to see it do well. Problem is, I'm from Yorkshire and I had a rule, if I didn't think a horse had shown enough ability to win a race after six weeks then it would have to go. Owners don't like that, but I'm not into bullshit!

That Newmarket yard was probably my favourite of all the ones I've owned or worked in. Yards are a funny thing you know, some are really lucky and it doesn't matter what trainer you have in there, you'll always get winners. Seriously. Other yards are completely the opposite and I've seen the best trainers brought down by a bad luck yard. Now, it may seem strange, but one of the key things to a successful yard is ventilation. Those old fashioned stables with their high ceilings were always the best. Cool in the summer and warm in winter, the horses never suffered from the bugs and infections you get in modern yards today.

For five years Janette and I made a real go of it and it is testament to another of Janette's attributes; she's not shy of hard work. However, it took a huge toll.

I was working eighteen-hour-days and so it should come as no surprise that in 2001 I had my first heart attack. We'd been out with friends in London and I'd driven home without any hold-ups. In fact it was the best drive out of London I've ever had and we got home around midnight. I remember feeling pretty unwell, bit of a tight chest, a pressing pain, but we went to bed. After a couple of hours I woke Janette to ask if she had any heartburn tablets. I thought I had bad indigestion. Thank goodness I woke her. She took one look at me and called an ambulance, although in my usual manner, I insisted I didn't need a doctor. If it wasn't for her persistence due to the seriousness of my heart attack I doubt very much that I would be here today, her quick thinking saved my life.

I was taken to hospital and given a barrage of tests and cardiograms. They were very concerned about my lack of oxygen and were panicking that my levels were so low. I was lying on an operating table and asked them why they had so many tubes in me. The doctor mentioned my oxygen levels and I said they'd been low since the cancer and the lung damage. Everyone sort of stopped moving around and at that point they sent me back up to intensive care where I would spend the next five days. In the morning they said they were sending for my medical records. Knowing the medical system the way that I did, I made a few calls and got hold of my records from the Royal Marsden. Not too sure why they couldn't just take my word for it, but as soon as they realised that it was indeed the damage from the chemo that was causing the issue the doctors relaxed quite a lot. I'd always known that my lung capacity was significantly affected, which is why I'd had to work so hard during recovery.

All of that said, it turned out a heart attack is quite a big deal. I was very ill and it really knocked me about. I couldn't walk for days, had no energy and it took a fair amount of time to get over it actually. Or it should have. I, of course, tried to get better too quickly. I can remember two weeks after the attack I went to do a job in Birmingham. Why? I don't know. Probably because I had been booked and didn't want to let anyone down. So off I went on my own. I managed to get through it somehow and driving home, nearly passed out. I pulled into a service station to try and rest but couldn't settle in the car so started driving again. Eventually I pulled in at a Little Chef and took a room there. I was simply too scared to go to sleep because I thought I was going to die, so after an hour of restless turning, I got back in the car and drove home. I really didn't help myself, so it took me a long time to get over the heart attack and to properly recover.

I think I must have come pretty close to dying, or maybe it was because my body was weakened by the chemo from years earlier, but I found it hard to come back. In the end we decided to sell the training yard. In hindsight, as much as I loved training, I finally had to admit that with everything else I was trying to do I could never give it the attention it deserved. Not being the best I could be meant that I didn't really have the passion for it. That and the simple fact, my passion was being focused elsewhere. The Trust had become too important for me not to give it my all. Although looking back, I couldn't have been too bad as one in seven of all my runners won.

We were incredibly fortunate to buy a beautiful old house previously owned by the greatest of all jockeys, Lester Piggott. I'll be honest, on moving in I did check the floor boards to see if Lester had left anything behind but I wasn't to be that lucky. I guess the taxman really did get the lot! We loved living there, bar one issue. Unfortunately it was during a time when night clubs were popular in Newmarket and with the house being in the dead centre of town it was just too noisy for us. After a couple of years we sold up and moved to Cheveley, a lovely village on the outskirts.

Just before the move we received the terrible news that Janette had breast cancer. During this time she was also helping to plan Sam and Ed's wedding as well as preparing the move and working fulltime. It all took its toll on her, but she never gave up and battled through to get everything done. I wish I could say that I handled this episode well, but I didn't. You'd think with my experience I'd have been the perfect companion, but for me it brought back all those awful memories and it scared me. Really scared me. I think having too much knowledge about a subject like cancer, can be worse than not knowing what is coming. I certainly wasn't the best person to help her go through it and basically wasn't there for her as I should have been and how you might think I would have been. Cancer affects people in so many different ways and for me it was a reminder that I couldn't face. Fortunately Janette responded well to treatment and has been cancer free for the last thirteen years. She is resilient in the extreme. Funnily enough though, if you asked her she'd probably tell you a different story. She may even say I gave her strength, but we're always hardest on ourselves.

I found the experience a sobering one. Cancer is indiscriminate and just because you've had it doesn't mean it won't touch another member of your family. Both my Mum and Dad passed away from this evil disease and Janette's daughter, Vicki is currently undergoing treatment, which saddens me enormously. You never know who it will come for next and this is why I am so passionate about fund raising. Being so involved with the Trust allows me the opportunity to hear how different people respond to the illness and to see a little of how my story has affected others. It's fascinating to me that I can have an impact on someone I've never met. Even now, people still come to me and tell me how I helped and inspired them. Recently Ed Chamberlain, ITV's new racing front man, recounted how he first reacted to me. It wasn't necessarily what I expected.

"Ah... I remember cursing Bob Champion for years. But, I should probably explain...

My grandfather loved the races and that's where I got my love of them from. Each National he'd let me pick a horse out and put a bet on for me. In 1981, aged seven, I'd chosen Spartan Missile. I remember being so excited in the final furlong as my horse was catching up to the leader, only to be beaten. I was furious that my horse had come in second, but of course I knew nothing of the enormity of what Bob had achieved. I also thought my jockey had given Spartan Missile a poor ride, again not knowing that John Thorne was a 54 year-old amateur and that both Bob and he had participated in one of the National's greatest fairy-tales. Of course as I grew up and discovered the real story of 1981, I was able to look back on the race with a completely different viewpoint from my much annoyed seven-year-old self.

I didn't actually know Bob whilst I was having my own cancer treatment in 2009, but to come back from cancer is one thing, to come back and win the National, wow that's incredible. I know that the differences in treatment from then to now are massive, but even so, mine was still brutal. Some days the chemo they put in me was so poisonous that it came in a red bag and you couldn't see the light through it. I'd take a couple of anti-sick pills and await the horrors I knew were coming. My incentive was always, every day to be well enough to get downstairs to WH Smiths in Southampton General Hospital and buy a copy of the Racing Post. If I could make it downstairs on my own then I knew I was going to be alright. It was racing that kept me going. I remember it was 2009 at Cheltenham and I was the first person in intensive care to have a television, admittedly it was also the Champions League that weekend too. AP McCoy had been great all through my journey with the treatment and I was devastated that he and Binocular didn't win the Champion Hurdle, but I got so excited when he won the Trophy Handicap Chase on Wichita Lineman that my drip came out of my arm. So I was really in trouble, not only did I have a TV, but I also had my drip hanging out of me. That's not a good thing in a cancer ward. I think they understood when I explained what a huge race it was. Possibly one of the greatest rides I've ever seen.

Heroes like Bob and at the time Lance Armstrong, were inspiring to me. Bob was a huge inspiration and you need inspirations like that when you're in hospital. Unlike Bob I wasn't tempted to pull any stunts with my drip to get out quicker and I left myself totally at the mercy of the hospital staff, who were incredible. I think Bob would say the same, that when you're going through treatment you crave being 'normal' again. You don't want any sympathy, you just want to walk down the street. I remember watching Bob's movie and seeing the late great John Hurt, when he's bald and hating the fact that he wasn't 'normal'. That's exactly what it's like. Even now, on a big day, I always have a quiet moment to reflect and think just how lucky I am. I imagine that Bob is the same. You don't look back and think it was so unfair, you just feel how lucky you are to have survived when so many aren't as fortunate."

Hearing Ed talk about Lance Armstrong made me think. It's so important when you're in the public eye to be someone that people look up to. Where cancer is involved then it's even more important to inspire and give hope. Initially I was very pleased to see what Lance Armstrong had achieved following our similar paths, so you can imagine my disappointment when the news was released regarding the drug taking. For me it would never have been a consideration and besides it wouldn't matter what I took, it wouldn't have made the horse run any faster! But I'm not trivialising what I understand would have been a need to compete at any cost. To me though this cost was too great and I felt he let those struggling with cancer down. I know he would have had a team behind him and they were probably as responsible as he was, but doing the right thing is always more important that winning.

In 2013, a couple of years after the trauma and anxiety of Janette being diagnosed, I had the additional ordeal of seeing Derek go through it too. Talking to him about it, he reminded me how he'd felt:

"I was absolutely knackered and could hardly get up and walk to the toilet. I remember asking Bob how he managed to win the National and he said something like, he was only thirty-years old at the time and completely fit, but for me, his survival was down to an inner strength that not many people see. We joke that he's only won the Grand National but having seen and then experienced myself what he went through, it's the most incredible thing.

When I was having my own treatment, the first time I walked into the chemo room everyone looked like they were dying and the sad part was that they may well have been. I'd known what Bob had gone through and thought, 'Well if Champs can get through it, so can I.' I was in Addenbrooke's Hospital and unlike most patients I wouldn't lie down. I would normally sit in a chair determined to prove to myself that I could and I would work as much as I could. One day I must have had a bad batch of chemo and I collapsed. I was very ill and three doctors rushed to take care of me. I woke up two hours later and there was Champs at the end of my bed. The first thing he said was, "You've caused a bit of excitement in here today."

I had no idea where I was and for a moment I thought I'd died and I'd gone to heaven and Bob was there and we were having a good laugh. It was only later that I learned he'd heard I'd collapsed and driven straight over to be there when I woke up. He'd chatted to other patients whilst I was being treated but had come in especially because he knew my wife had to do the school run. I was just so stunned that he was there.

He would say that he isn't good to help anyone going through cancer but he is, having beaten it, he gives you the impetus and forthrightness to go forward. He was exactly like that with me as well as Janette. He's not a cuddly man, but he'll push you to get up so that you can get on. He went through it 1981 and even now, almost forty years later, people still come up to him and say thank you for giving me hope or for helping my mother and he is never blasé because he truly understand the importance of hope."

It's a very humbling thing to hear your friend talk of you in that way and I am glad I am still around to hear it, because ten years to the exact day and almost the exact hour since I had my first heart attack, I had a second. This time I knew the symptoms. I rang Mary and she told me to get to the hospital and stop messing about. I did and they got me straight in and added another stent. This episode didn't knock me about as much as the first, but the infection I contracted afterwards was far worse than the actual attack. What we do know is that the attacks are a result of the chemotherapy. The doctors had warned me that this could happen and of the patients that had the same treatment at the same time as me, many have had heart attacks and not survived. The problem is that the drugs damaged a lot of blood vessels around the heart. Thankfully, I've been fine since with no further heart problems.

φ

However whilst my heart may physically have been fine, in 2010 it was to shatter as Mum passed away aged 90. You've probably gathered by now that I was very much a mum's boy and I loved her dearly. She wasn't to have the same mercy as my Dad as she became very ill with bone cancer. Now no cancer is good, but bone cancer is agony and she suffered horribly for months. There was nothing we could do except watch her becoming more and more frail. Mary was with her daily and I was there as often as I could be. I would have done anything to take away her pain and it broke me to see her trying to be strong for us. I know that this sounds harsh but Mary would say the same, towards the end, in her last few days it would have been kinder to have helped her slip away. We show far more compassion to animals than we ever do to those we love. Sadly, but mercifully, on the 2nd October 2010, she died. Mary rang me that morning and I jumped in the car and drove there as fast as I could. I arrived just in time before they took her away and I was able to say my goodbyes.

Mary and I were bereft, but life must go on. That afternoon Mary had to put on her robes as Mayoress of Wootton Bassett and carry out her Civic Service Duty. At the time there were a lot of military repatriations coming through the area from RAF Lyneham and the services were so important. I know Mary didn't really want to go and I don't think anyone would have thought less of her for it, but we could both hear Mum telling us not to be daft and to carry on. Mary was praying that no one would mention it but of course they did and it was so hard for her to do what she had to. I was incredibly proud of the inner strength she showed that day.

I'd already scattered Dad's ashes on Roseberry Topping, a local landmark in the North Yorkshire Moors and close to our old family home. We all agreed to do the same for Mum. On the day though I had a terrible chest infection and shouldn't have been out of bed let alone climbing a 320m hill. I really did try my best, but had to admit defeat halfway up, so Mary, Emma and Nick climbed to the top to scatter her ashes. I can't forgive myself for not being there, but whenever I get the chance I climb to the top and talk to them both. I share my thoughts and let them know that they're still with me. I miss my Mum every day, she was the real, true constant in my life. Like all mothers she loved unconditionally and mine had a heart as big as Yorkshire. Mary has now become the one that receives my phone calls at least three times a day and whilst Mum can't be replaced, Mary is a pretty close second in my affections. Just don't tell her I said that!

In 2011 I was finding that I had some spare time on my hands and as if I'd requested something to fill it, I was offered a job doing speaking gigs on cruise ships. Not something I'd initially considered, but my goodness what a lot of fun. I worked on almost forty ships over a five year period and met some incredible people, including making firm friends with celebrities like Roy Walker and Des O'Connor.

The very first cruise I did was a sports themed trip on the QE2 with a whole bunch of famous sportsmen and women, Willie Thorne, my former suffering golf companion and Colin Jackson, the sprint hurdler, were with me and it was such a fun time, even though I was seasick. After that first one I started to get asked to do more and what was better, they offered to pay me for it. All in all, quite the deal. Paid cruising.

The ships travelled to places such as Australia, Japan, Hawaii, Fiji and the Caribbean. We always had nice cabins and were discouraged from going below decks to mix with the crew. We all ignored this of course as they were very friendly and we enjoyed spending time with them when off duty. You had to be on your best behaviour, any improper behaviour would mean that you'd be off the ship and wouldn't be booked again. For some of the single men it meant turning down a lot of offers from bored wives.

I always chose to work the adult only ships. Not because I have anything against children, but I think being trapped on board a ship with too many screaming kids might have made me go overboard!

Of course being paid, we were expected to do several shows during the time away. I remember my first ever one. I got up on stage and delivered what I considered to be my best speech. Afterwards, feeling really pleased with myself, I bumped into Rod Taylor. He had worked as a comedian and in later life a producer for Granada TV, working on talent shows. Rod spent his time on the cruises talking about his days in TV, a subject I thought far more interesting than anything I had to say.

Well, he pulled me aside and said, "That was alright Bob. Well done."

"Thanks."

"What are you going to say the next two times?"

I looked at him blankly and asked, "What do you mean?"

He smiled. "You do know that you have to give three talks don't you?"

I hadn't realised that and had used up all my best material in that first one! He told me that he would spend time with me that very day to help me plan my talks. In fact he spent a lot of time with me working on them and invested a great deal of his own expertise. He was the biggest help to my speaking career I could ever have had. I can't thank him enough for that. We got it sorted so that I would do two speeches and then a Q&A for the last one and it worked really well. Rod did tell me that it didn't always go well for him either and on his very first TV appearance, doing a weather forecast, three quarters of the way through the broadcast all of the weather icons that he had stuck to the board fell off. It took a little bit of his comedic talent to get him out of it and after that he decided he'd be better off being a producer.

On returning from that first paid trip out, I went to see Rod in his then home town of Alderley Edge. We met early in the morning at the café above the library and he sat us by the window, saying that it would be quite a sight for me. Sure enough it was school dropping-off time and all of the Premier League footballers' wives and girlfriends (the WAGs) turned up in their Range Rovers, all beautifully dressed and done up. It was quite a spectacle I can tell you, but that wasn't all. Rod and I spent the day together in the café and over the course of it the same women appeared like clockwork for the gym, the hairdressers and finally school pick-up, each time in a completely different outfit! What a totally removed lifestyle they lead. I've mixed with some very well off people in my time, but I've never seen such an obvious show of money in my life.

Thankfully Rod was great company and ran a really funny commentary throughout. I think the WAG lifestyle must be exhausting. I grumble about having to get changed into a suit once a day!

Given the types of celebrities the cruise companies were using, the one thing that was noticeably absent were egos. No one was too full of themselves and if you did have an attitude it was knocked out of you fairly quickly! To be honest though it was quite a lonely lifestyle whilst on board. During the day you would walk around and mingle with the guests and personally I would eat little and often. It was a good way to lose weight, although I did end up drinking more than I normally would, partially out of being sociable. I think that if I lived on cruise ships I'd become a quite high-end functioning alcoholic as there is so much drink available and it's encouraged. In the afternoon you'd go and watch a movie and maybe take in a show then get ready for dinner. I also went to the gym everyday just to stay in some sort of shape.

It didn't take too long to learn the ropes and the 'cruise etiquette'. We would sit at dinner each night on our allotted tables and talk politely with the guests. We were assigned tables and these were 'our guests' to entertain. Often we'd double-up on a table to provide a bit of support or light relief for each other. In the evening we'd attend a show to support our fellow entertainers and then it was time for our favourite activity; the quiz nights. Although we weren't allowed to win, we'd still get quite competitive with our teams. Often we'd already know the questions but we'd join in with the guests to help them to success. We had some really good laughs on those nights. However it wasn't always fun and I remember on one cruise, my allotted table was full of attendees from a stamp collecting convention. They were lovely people, but a little obsessed about their hobby. Now I knew nothing about stamps but my goodness by the end of that trip I knew more than I ever wanted to! Ask me now and the only bit of trivia I can remember is that the Penny Black isn't the most expensive stamp. Sadly, I can't tell you what is! On that voyage I did make friends with the head waiter so I got the heads up as to what was being served for dinner. I'd arrive at the very last moment, place my order and then precisely forty-three minutes later I'd have to excuse myself to help out with the evening's entertainment. It might not sound like a lot but when you are surrounded by a table of extremely keen philatelists, forty-three minutes can drag by like you wouldn't believe.

My favourite person to be on-board with was Martin Daniels, the magician Paul Daniels' son. What a showman! You could see that his Dad had taught him well and Debbie Magee was a tremendous dancer. She had a stage presence all of her own. Such a talented family.

Of course the comedians were always well received and I used to love sitting with Des O'Connor. He was so funny and I was lucky to become firm friends with both him and Martin over the years. One of the other surprise bonuses when it came to friendship was that if I was travelling to Australia I used the opportunity to meet up with Ken Hunt. He'd retired there to be with his daughter and when we stopped in harbour, he'd pick me up and we'd spend the day together. It was always such a pleasure. We still spoke weekly on the telephone and always had time to catch up.

I soon picked up a reputation as the 'WiFi' man on board. Anyone who knows me knows that I am lost without an Internet connection and so I made it my mission to find the best WiFi signal on the ships. WiFi on a cruise ship is expensive, that's a fact, and being 'staff' didn't mean they let you have it any cheaper, so I thought it was crucial that you got the best signal and therefore your money's worth. Yes, I am northern and proud. At times I felt like the WiFi Pied Piper as I would have staff and guests following me on the hunt for the elusive sweet spot. They just knew I'd find the best place to get a strong signal. After a couple of cruises I figured out that the best and most efficient use of the signal was to write all of my emails and messages in advance and then as soon as I found the signal I could just press send. That one little trick saved me a fortune. I also wouldn't read anything then and there, I'd just download it to read later. It's these little things that made me smile and I considered them a win, albeit a trivial one.

On the first few trips I'd go on shore whenever we docked and I got to see some beautiful sights. It was totally different to promoting the movie, here I had time to sightsee. I've been so lucky to visit some of the most amazing places in the world. I think the

Peterhof Palace, in St Petersburg, Russia is one of the most stunning things I've seen. It just hits you, not only the architecture but the whole feel of the place, the history and the grandeur, it's entirely different to any other part of St Petersburg. Of course, after a few trips the thought of queuing yet again with thousands of other tourists takes the shine off and you tend to avoid the more populated sights. Still, there are so many different things that stick in my mind. The undaunted cheerfulness of those in the Caribbean, despite having very little in the way of wealth, they would always greet you with a smile and were so friendly, the stunning views of Honolulu and the quiet tranquillity of the Norwegian Fjords. Also Hiroshima was such an interesting place. Not somewhere you'd automatically think about visiting, but I was fascinated by it. It was both beautiful in the way it had been rebuilt and knowing what had happened there, very moving too. I also loved Tallinn in Estonia, what a gorgeous town and I was lucky enough to go there several times. I recall once when we docked there they were hosting the World Netball Championship. I don't think I have ever seen so many fit women in one place and their legs! Oh my goodness they went on forever. Well, I suppose you have to be tall to play netball! I stayed on the ship and watched the tournament from there but I don't think there is a better combination in life than a beautiful city, beautiful sport and beautiful women!

Of course being me, again it wasn't all plain sailing. I had to have a little dodgy run in with my mortality. I'm not a good swimmer, in fact I can just about do a few lengths, but one day whilst visiting New Zealand, for some strange reason I decided to go swimming in the sea. Perhaps it was the beautiful yet empty beach, with not a soul in sight. Perhaps it was the sun and the light breeze, perhaps it was the water reflecting off the gentle waves, perhaps it was because I had taken leave of my senses. Whatever the reason, I saw a small secluded island with trees and thought I'd paddle my way over. You hear about rip tides and you see them in movies, but it isn't until you get caught in one that you realise just how strong and scary they really are. I wasn't in too deep, only probably up to my shoulders and suddenly I felt something pulling at me, tugging me down and sideways. It was very strong, like what I'd imagine a big, heavy-set rugby player tackling you would feel like. I thought I'd best go back and I was fortunate to get away with it. Of course the solitude of the place had meant that if I hadn't got back, no one would have been around to fish me out! You'd think after that scary encounter I'd have learnt my lesson but no, whilst in the Caribbean I did the same thing. Fortunately I'd been reading about the riptides in the local waters and knew what was happening so I got out pretty smart'ish. Again, I was very lucky as apparently there had been quite a few deaths of tourists caught out that way.

On another trip we were heading from New Zealand to Sydney, Australia. Unlike what you might think, they aren't really that close to one another. In fact there's more than 2000km of the Tasman Sea lying between them. One night, halfway across to Australia, I woke up and thought how quiet it was. Then I realised that the ship had stopped. That was unusual. Not only had it stopped but clearly the stabilisers were off and the ship was rolling slightly. Obviously we'd broken down and so my brain got to work. I remember thinking that it would take a tug boat a week to get to us and to tow us to harbour so I figured we'd definitely have enough food and probably enough water. But what really concerned me was that I had a job to get to back home and my schedule was pretty tight as it was. I suppose that just about sums me up. My greatest fear about being broken down in the middle of the ocean, with the potential of drifting off to goodness knows where, was that I'd be late for another appointment! Thankfully though the Ship's engineers got us back underway after only a few hours.

One of the last cruises I did was to Saint Martin. It was a lovely port and sometimes would have up to twenty-six cruise liners visiting on any one day, with thousands of tourists roaming around the place. It was a very beautiful spot and the locals were always so friendly. I was really saddened to see the news recently about how the island had been devastated by hurricane Irma.

To get home from the cruises they would fly you up to the nearest main airport hub. Leaving Saint Martin I was to fly to Fort Lauderdale and on settling into the plane I noticed that the first two seats were taken up by engineers. Never a good sight on any plane when you're about to take off!

We got to the end of the runway and the plane died, so the engineers got off and tried to fix it. They must have known the aircraft had problems for the engineers to be on board. That didn't give me much confidence. So we sat on the plane for an hour but it wasn't going to go. There were a hundred or so passengers and finally they carted us back to the airport. We spent a few hours waiting to see what would happen and eventually they said they'd found us a hotel. They were providing buses, but I took one look at the queue and decided that wasn't for me. I grabbed a taxi with about eight other people and our suitcases. It was a bit of a squeeze and I ended up with two women sat on my lap in the front seat. Well we made it to the hotel only to be told that they were fully booked! I don't know why but I was nominated as spokesperson for our little group and went over to try to explain that the airport had sent us. They kept telling me that they were fully booked. I looked around and it made no sense, the place was empty and the airport had specifically told us this was the hotel to go to. I went back and forth between the group and the reception until finally, I demanded to know where their guests were if they were fully booked? The receptionist told me straight that they were expecting over a hundred guests coming from the airport. I felt like I was in some strange outtake of Fawlty Towers. If it hadn't been so frustrating I'd probably have laughed but I eventually got them to realise that we were the advance party that had come to the hotel from the airport. Finally we got booked in. End of drama? Not a chance. The next day we were to be trooped back to the airport and of course I didn't want to wait for everyone else so I took myself off again. I got to customs first only to be told that I'd already left according to my passport. I explained again what had happened, that we had gone through customs but never left the island but they weren't convinced and thought that I either had a fake passport or was up to no good. Finally after about an hour of explaining, they let me through. I parted with the comment that there was another hundred people like me on the way, so they had better get their act together.

Some of my least favourite cruise trips were the ones that took us across the Bay of Biscay. I can tell you now it's not a pleasant run and I was often very seasick. Mother Nature will be Mother

Nature and in the Bay, if she's in the mood for it, she'll have the seas pounding and the waves sky high. You knew it was going to be a bad one when the storm clouds came rolling in. At times the weather would be so atrocious that the crews couldn't serve food, not that anyone wanted to eat it anyway! I'm assured that it's not always that bad, but to be honest I've never had a good crossing of that Bay and it's one route I'd never sail again.

The last cruise I did was for Saga Cruises on the MS Saga Ruby in the first months of 2013. This was going to be the ship's last sailing and we were heading off to the Caribbean when one of the generators failed, disabling the ship's air-conditioning plant. We were stuck in the Azores for two days and then the company decided to cancel the original itinerary and sail through the Med instead. It offered the passengers a chance to get off and have their money refunded although many stayed on-board. I felt so sorry for the guests that remained as they all had their summer clothes with them and now we were heading into winter in Europe. It was a shame to end my time on the cruises that way and I wondered if maybe I'd killed the ship! The thing is, these massive vessels have so many things that can go wrong and at least we hadn't broken down on the high seas. Just to round my final trip off, on the way home we went back through the Bay of Biscay and yes, it was as rough as ever.

I think I'd consider doing the whole 'cruise ship talks' again, but I'd have to choose the locations. It was nice to be away and I could relax in the foreign cities as I rarely got recognised.

φ

Being recognised in the UK is a fairly constant thing for me now and for the vast majority of the time it is lovely. Who doesn't like people coming up and wishing you well and congratulating you on what you've done. It's such a nice thing to happen and of course for the most part it is very informal. But in 2011, I was to be recognised in a much more formal way and I must say it is one of the proudest moments of my life.

Having received the 1981 BBC Sports Personality Team of the Year Award, you can imagine my total surprise at being told, some thirty years later, that I had won the BBC Sports Personality Helen Rollason Award. It is given for 'outstanding achievement in the face of adversity', and was recognising the work done by the Trust and how much we had raised to that point.

I do consider it to be one of my biggest achievements in life and I was truly honoured and humbled to receive such a prestigious award, especially as it is named after a ground-breaking sports journalist who herself had sadly succumbed to cancer.

I would like to say that having been given advance notice for the evening I was prepared and ready for it. I wasn't. I'm not sure how I got through my speech because I was absolutely petrified, it was far scarier than any race I'd ever ridden in. I didn't want to cock it up in front of all my family and friends who were there, let alone the small matter of the sixteen million television viewers watching.

One of the simplest sounding, yet hardest, things to do was to walk down the entrance way to the stage in the correct amount of time. They told me that they'd call my name out and then they would play a piece of pre-recorded video film and I shouldn't arrive on stage too early. I managed it, just about. The video they showed was terrific in itself, because they had edited together footage of actual races and excerpts from the film, 'Champions' and some other old interviews and special footage of cancer cells. The whole thing had a fantastic voiceover recorded by John Hurt. Talk about being made to feel special. Add to that the whole audience, filled with amazing sports stars, decided to give me an impromptu standing ovation as I approached the stage. It was extremely emotional. Topping it all off, was the fact that the trophy was formally presented to me by AP McCoy, the most successful jump jockey ever. Quite fittingly he was sporting the cuts and bruises that are the mark of a National Hunt jockey on his face that night.

I managed to keep myself together, but if you look back at the clip you'll see I'm quite choked up. I know that what I said was all from the heart because I hadn't prepared any remarks or a speech. I thought that if I just said how I felt it would be the best thing and people tell me it came out alright. I can't tell you if it did or not, as I never watch anything that I'm in other than old races. I have it all on tape but can't bring myself to view it. I get embarrassed, I think I've got a terrible voice and I don't like listening to myself. If I do ever hear any recordings back I think, 'What did you say that for?' even if I haven't said anything stupid. Although I trust my family and friends and they reported that my Helen Rollason acceptance speech was very good and that's kind of them. I do remember that I was able to thank all the people I wanted to, but especially Mary and my friend Josh Gifford. I mentioned how, when I had been written off and everyone was saying that I was finished, he had stood by me. No one knew that just two short months later he would be taken from us by a heart attack. How fortunate I was to be able to thank him that night.

Henri recalls:
> *"It was a fantastic event, we were backstage waiting and it was arranged with almost military precision. All Dad's close friends and family, including Janette and me, and Derek and so many others were all there. We had to file onto the stage whilst the video was being shown and whilst Dad walked to the stage. There was a huge audience, and I don't think I'd properly realised just how much people were aware of what he'd achieved until the standing ovation. It wasn't scripted. It just happened. It was such an emotional moment for us all being there."*

One other highlight of that night was that it took place in the presence of Her Royal Highness Anne, The Princess Royal, a fantastic horsewoman herself. As I've said before, over the years I have been privileged to spend time with members of the Royal Family, mainly the Queen Mother, whom I respected enormously and who if I'm honest was basically just like a mum. That's the only way I can describe her. She was someone who made you feel comfortable in her presence and had such a gentle manner.

I've also been fortunate enough to have met Her Majesty The Queen many times since she presented me with my MBE and she has always been extremely friendly and generous. Recently, on a trip to Paris, I was sitting next to her at a dinner engagement on

behalf of the Trust and I was very impressed by Her Majesty's ability to speak French. I hadn't really considered it before, but she is
fluent and very lucky for me as I don't speak a word and she very
graciously spared my ignorance by telling me what was being said!
The Queen is a very down to earth lady who rarely forgets anyone
and who will chat at length about horses, in that way she is very
similar to her mother. I often think it's easy to forget that beneath
everything else they are people who have loves and hobbies just
like us.

As you may imagine, beyond an appropriate deference, I'm
not one for airs and graces. This can occasionally cause me to say
things a bit more bluntly than perhaps I should. In 2013 I was
kindly invited to travel to Ascot in one of the Royal carriages which
is a huge honour and Janette and I were thrilled. Janette loves the
opportunity to get dressed up and I certainly don't mind the odd bit
of formal style. On arriving at Ascot I saw Princess Anne. His
Royal Highness, Prince Philip was unfortunately unwell and in
hospital at the time and me being me, I simply asked, "How's your
father?"

As soon as the words were out, it dawned on me I should
probably have referred to him by his proper title, but Princess Anne
is such a lovely, straight talking lady that she replied, "He's much
better thanks and will sometimes do anything to get out of racing!"

I guess it's a good thing they know I mean no harm and am
just a plain talking Yorkshire man meaning no disrespect.

The work of the Trust was given a real boost by the Helen
Rollason award and I was continuing to drive the length and
breadth of the country attending talks and conferences and charity
events. Add to that my normal personal travel and I imagine some
weeks, even now, I might do over 1,000miles on the road. Most of
the journeys are uneventful, but in March 2015 I was to come as
close to death as any heart attack or cancer had brought me.

I was tootling along the M11 and having a good run for once
after being to see Jonjo O'Neill. The traffic began to slow and then,
as is the way of motorways in the UK, for no reason it came to a
complete stop. One rule that I have when driving and something I
have always done, is to keep a large gap between myself and any

cars stopping ahead of me. It's seen me right on many an occasion. On this particular day it saved my life.

Coming up the last hill on the M11 before my turn-off I saw the cars ahead coming to a stop. I slowed down and maintained my usual large gap in front. I had only been stationary for a few seconds when I was hit from behind. The car that went into me was being driven by an off-duty police officer who had also stopped, but was himself rear-ended by a campervan. My car was shunted forward, but because of the gap I had left, I didn't get crushed into the vehicle in front of me. There is no doubt it made all the difference when compared to the carnage behind me.

The police officer had his children in the back of his car and luckily they had been saved by their car seats. The officer though was not so fortunate. I knew by the colour of him that he wasn't going to make it. There was so much blood and he was just sitting, strapped into his seat with the car squashed around him. It was horrendous to watch him slowly die, trapped in the car. By the time the paramedics got to him it was too late to save him. I felt so sorry for those poor children.

We were stuck on the M11 for hours and my car was a write off. The attending police breathalysed me as routine but as I never drink and drive that wasn't a problem. Yet the rest of the measures they put me through would have made you think I'd caused the accident rather than just being stationary. They took my phone to see if I was texting or talking on it, even though I wasn't moving at the actual time of the impact. It was quite an eye opener really as I know people think that if they're stopped in their car then it's okay to check messages. This isn't the case and I could have been prosecuted for not paying attention. Luckily for me I always use Bluetooth when driving and so there were no issues. It still took six days to get my phone back, and that was after calling in a favour to help me recover it.

The driver of the van was sentenced to three years for driving without due care and attention and I realised quite starkly that it only takes a second to be distracted, yet in that second so much devastation and loss can happen. I was lucky enough to only suffer from minor whiplash but the effect on me mentally has lingered and whilst I still drive over 1,000miles each week, I'm not as happy behind the wheel as I once was.

It's been said that I've had a charmed yet difficult life and I think they could be right. I must have a Guardian Angel. I can't paint or draw but if you asked me today I could paint the face of that poor police officer as he quietly died on a motorway for no reason. I recall it so clearly.

I've mentioned already that I'd ban tractors off the roads. Maybe this uneasiness in driving now is why, if I ever did have any influence over such things, I'd introduce a lot of changes. Derek laughs at me when I go on a rant, but as well as a 7am to 10pm tractor ban, lorries would not be allowed to overtake, ever! Cyclists... well probably best not to get me started on them, suffice to say they'd all have to have insurance for a start! It might seem that I'm a moaning old git but driving the amount I do, I know the delays all three of them cause me. Of course I am well aware that this makes me a complete hypocrite, as back when I was a lad I used to drive tractors on the road and nothing gave me greater pleasure than to see a long winding trail of cars behind me! Perhaps all the delays I get caught up in now are payback for me holding up other drivers as a boy. Funnily enough that reminds me of an incident way back when I was probably only fifteen and the pin snapped between the tractor I was driving and its trailer. The trailer became unhitched and, full of bales of hay, hurtled down the hill to a main road. I was trying to head it off on the tractor but had no chance. It ploughed through a fence and luckily for me, flew between two cars and landed in a ditch on its side. That was such a busy road and I was terrified it would kill someone. Had it been today with the amount of traffic on the road it would have hit a car without a doubt.

When I'm driving I tend to listen to BBC Radio 2. My favourite way of passing a half hour is listening to Pop Master with Ken Bruce. Now, obviously you'd think that with the amount of time I'm in the car listening to the radio and with the years creeping up on me, I'd be pretty good... I'm not! My average score is one and my personal best is four, so I don't see me entering anytime soon. I do like music though and back in 1988 I had the great privilege of being on the BBC's Desert Island Discs with Sue Lawley.

I had to choose eight records, a book and a luxury item. The book I chose was 'Fraser's Horse Book – The Complete Book of Horse Care' by Alistair Fraser and Frank Manolson. Not too sure what use it was going to be for me on a desert island with presumably no horses, but I took it anyway because once I'd read it I could have saved quite a lot on vet's bills. The luxury item was a bronze statue of Aldaniti jumping Becher's, sculpted by the former jockey Philip Blacker (who had finished third to us on Royal Mail). I just loved it as a thing of beauty to look at and still do.

As for the music, I chose the tracks at the time for a whole range of reasons and I might well change my mind on some of them nowadays, but most of them are still favourites. There was 'If I Were a Carpenter' by the Four Tops and 'Happy Christmas' by John Lennon. For obvious reasons I picked the theme music from the movie 'Champions' and added to that was the Rolling Stones 'Satisfaction', Rod Stewart's 'Sailing', and Glen Campbell's, 'Galveston'. My favourite choice was Simon and Garfunkel's 'Bridge over Troubled Water' and I still think it is the best record ever made. Maybe it is the theme tune for my life.

Speaking of life, as I mentioned earlier in the book, I was declared dead on Wikipedia! It took me six months to get 'resurrected'. I only found out about it when a client rang to see if I was still alive and was okay to do the presentation I was booked for. I would never have thought how difficult it is to reclaim your life once they've killed you off! So that was the second time, as Mark Twain would have said, 'Reports of my death are greatly exaggerated.' I keep telling people, I have no plans to go just yet, so they can all wait a while. I'm just being happy with life as it is.

I'm not too busy to help out where I can though and Mary often calls upon me to help with events close to her heart.

Over the last few years, Bob has become a great friend to us all at the Royal Wootton Bassett Town Council.

When Bob visits his sister Mary, he often pops in the council office to see us for a chat over a cuppa and his favourite chocolate biscuits.

In 2016 his sister Mary was Mayor of Royal Wootton

Bassett and invited Bob to be the guest of honour at our Christmas Event to switch on the lights. Bob agreed, even though he knew he would be cutting it fine, having to travel from London.

He made it just in time and appeared on stage to a massive crowd gathered on the High Street, who warmly welcomed him switching on the lights.

It was a great honour for our Town having Bob do this for us.

Michelle Temple

I've become quietly fond of Royal Wootton Bassett as it's now so deservedly known.

Today, Janette and I have a lovely home in Newmarket. Unfortunately, due to her job in London and my charity work and personal speaking events, at times it could seem like we are ships passing in the night. However, we always talk several times during the day and we ensure that when we are together the time is exclusively ours. After all these years we are extremely happy and content.

Although on a recent special birthday for Janette I almost ended up lynched! We'd gone on holiday to Florida with her daughters, Sam and Vicki, and I mentioned that the four of us had been invited to a Christmas party at a friend of a friend's house in Port Royal; an exclusive part of town. I insisted it would be a very smart affair but the girls had only packed casual clothes, so they decided to go on a shopping trip at considerable expense for black dresses, shoes etc. However, when we arrived at the party it was certainly not what I had anticipated. It was very casual, we felt extremely overdressed and of course it was all my fault, having not listened to the details of the invitation properly. We made our excuses, left early and instead had dinner in our favourite restaurant by the dockside, so at least they had one reason to be all dressed up.

I always liked Florida as a holiday destination, despite that disaster Ian Watkinson and I had all those years ago and I liked it mainly for the sunshine and warmth. There's very little I hate but cold damp weather would be top of my list. Yes, I know I live in the wrong country to hate that, but some days I wake up in agony and the cold and damp only ever makes it worse. It's not just me, a lot of us old jockeys do and I presume it's because of the damage we did in the many falls we suffered. I guess it's probably a touch of arthritis in the joints and it plays up. Cold and damp days are my bug bears. When it's miserable like that I do wonder at the things I've put myself through, but I head off for a sauna and tell myself to stop moaning. Although I'm sure I probably whinge a bit to Janette.

When asked how she's put up with me all these years, Janette says quite simply:

Living with Bob, can sometimes be challenging, he has a wicked sense of humour and at times, being from York-shire, he doesn't realise how his words can be taken, but I am quite patient and have just learned to let things go. Bob is a caring and supportive partner, he can be slightly impatient if you are late and dislikes getting into traffic jams, but he is a lot more "chilled" than he used to be! Another dislike is that he never relishes the prospect of waiting in for a delivery or tradesperson, who only give a morning or afternoon time slot. He cannot comprehend why they cannot give a definite time. He is definitely obsessed with mowing the lawn, which has to be done to perfection.

Since being together for the past twenty years, we have had numerous obstacles to overcome, but together we have done this, and our relationship is even stronger.

I am extremely proud of his achievements and passion for fund raising for his Cancer Trust. During the years we have visited many amazing places in the UK and abroad where we have met some lovely and interesting people. There have been so many highlights but one occasion which was very special was when we were VIP Guests of Honour at the Ascot Racing Carnival in Perth Australia. We were picked up by helicopter at the hotel, given an amazing tour of the city, and then flown directly into the racecourse.

I don't think Bob will ever retire as he likes to keep busy, although I do feel that occasionally he drives himself too hard, to the point of exhaustion.

So we are happy together when spending time in one another's company, but she probably doesn't enjoy watching TV with me as I love being in control of the 'doofer'. I think that I can multitask and watch several programmes at once, but in reality I'm most likely really annoying with it and am a flicker of the worst order. It takes quite a programme to stop me and hold my attention and I suppose my favourite would be Countryfile. Not a real surprise given that I grew up in the beautiful rural settings of Yorkshire and am still a country boy at heart. I try to watch the programme when I can and it definitely has the only useful weather forecast out of all of them, even if they glamorise farming and country living. I also like most nature documentaries, again probably no big surprise there, but what might shock you is my other television loves. I enjoy nothing more than tuning into the US crime shows like NCIS and CSI. Obviously I try to guess whodunit, but mainly I am fascinated by the science of forensics.

As I am thinking about my likes and dislikes here, I realise that although I used to be a fan of Corrie and Emmerdale, after a while I drifted away from them. I suppose I realised that you can only have so many deaths or plane crashes in one place before people would move out. I mean, would you keep going to the Woolpack if you thought every passenger plane overhead was going to come into the lounge bar? They've just stopped being as realistic and grounded as they once were.

I'm going to admit to a guilty pleasure and it's Strictly Come Dancing. Yes, yes I know, it's not the done thing for a gruff Yorkshire man to admit to, but I really love it. You'd never get me on it though as I have someone else's two left feet when it comes to dancing. Seriously, I am hopeless and I don't care how good the professional dancers are, they'd never get me to look good. I was a judge once on the old 'Come Dancing' up in Blackpool, although why I was is a bit beyond my recollection. It would be like asking

Wayne Sleep to be the starter at the Grand National. He could do it, but it would be a strange combination. I really had no clue but luckily the professionals went first with their scores and I just went higher or lower by one so that I looked like I knew what I was saying. I think that professional dancers on 'Strictly' are amazing and truly talented in the way that they can choreograph a dance and help the 'star' look good. Anyone who goes on it has my utmost respect.

Aside from the occasional TV show, I don't tend to relax much. I find it really hard to switch off, but I sometimes watch movies and these can help me wind down at the end of the day. I've always enjoyed a good western and it takes me back to the days of being a boy with Howard and Derek, shooting at the bad guys from the sofa! My favourite film will always be the Magnificent Seven, what an absolute classic. I can't tell you how many times I've seen it but I'll always watch it when it's on.

I know that in general I can be pretty frustrating to be around as I constantly pace about. I have a lot of pent up energy to burn off. Janette I think is mostly used to it by now, but it does drive her mad on occasion and I often hear. "Bob! For goodness sake, sit down!"

Even in the night I am restless. I don't sleep all that well and I'm often awake between 2am and 4am. A few years ago I would have slept in every bed in the house just to try to settle but I don't tend to do that now. Perhaps it's because I spend so much of my day sitting down in the car, perhaps I'm not exercising enough or maybe I'm just not willing to give in to sleep.

That all sounds like I'm living a terribly restless life, but I'm not. I love life and one thing that is especially terrific is that because I no longer have to waste like a jockey, I have a deep and passionate love affair with food. Sweet stuff especially. I've been known to skip courses and have two puddings. My Mum's trifle was always my favourite and even though I know they're simple to make, she had something about hers that was very special and I do miss them. I have to make do with meringues which are another favourite. If I'm feeling really naughty in the morning then it's a bacon butty for breakfast, but I hope Janette doesn't read this bit or I'll be in trouble.

She and Mary are constantly on to me to give up fizzy drinks. Apparently they're bad for my health, but having got this far I think that I'm alright and I basically ignore the nagging! That said, on a recent cancer check-up my bloods had a poor result and they were concerned for a time. They asked me to come back for another test a week later. I laid off the fizzy drinks in the interim and strangely enough the test results were much better. Still a man has to have a vice and anyway, I need the energy to help me with my one main obsession in life.

Anyone who follows me on Facebook will know that when I am not off at the races or giving speeches for the Trust, I mow lawns. I mean, I mow lawns a lot! It probably comes from my days of ploughing on the farm, but I am incredibly particular about my lines having to be straight and not just 'sort of' straight. I mean plumbline straight. Winning ploughing competitions taught me how to follow a line and I will mark both ends of a long garden to make sure I get things looking proper. I'd be fuming if I messed up. Thinking about it, that's the thing that really makes me unwind. I get a deep sense of satisfaction and it keeps my hands busy whilst my mind turns off the clutter and focuses on the task.

I do get teased about it quite a bit on Facebook by my friends but I'll cope and I love the way social media has united and reunited me with so many of my friends that otherwise I might not see for months or even years at a time. I feel incredibly lucky to have made so many friends over the years and have been rewarded with their loyalty and their trust. Sally and Nigel Dimmer, who'll you remember gave me the Aintree horseshoe, have been constants in my life for almost forty years and it's great that I am still able to see them regularly. When I said I was writing a book, Sally thought she'd share some stories, but only if I promised to put them in, unabridged. Well, I couldn't say no really, and as it turns out, they're not as bad or as embarrassing as they could have been.

"We met Bob through Bob Davies the night before his first biopsy and we've been friends ever since. We no longer have a guest room we have, 'Bob's room' as he's stayed in it so often. He really is part of our family and we love him to bits. Over the years we've been with him through so many different parts of his life. He's usually late for dinner, especially if he's out with Nigel, as they often take the Cheltenham Gold Cup round to local hotels and I can guarantee they'll arrive back late. He also has to be excused between courses so that he can check his phone which is infuriating."

I did think she was going to tell about the memorable occasion when Nigel and I ended up in a Cheltenham lap dancing club! So I should probably add it in here for completeness. The owners and girls of the club had decided to do a fund raising event for the Trust, which was very kind of them and Nigel and I went to collect a cheque. Now I am not quite sure why, but somehow we managed to lose track of time and almost missed dinner! My goodness we got a rollicking from Sally for that one, especially when my plea of, "It's for charity" was proven a bit false when the club went bust a few days later and the cheque bounced.

Sally says:

"Bob does love women and this has gotten him into lots of trouble. We had a cook working for us who was a terribly pretty girl. Bob popped into the kitchen to chat to her and I followed him in.

"Leave the poor girl alone Champion," I said and she looked up at the mention of his name.

"Are you 'the' Bob Champion?" she asked.

He puffed out his chest a little and said in his best debonair voice, "I was the last time I looked."

She gave him such a sweet smile and said, "My Dad used to date your ex-wife Jo!"

He scurried out of the kitchen and obviously took the time to come up with a suitable funny line. When she came in with the first course he said cheekily, "I bet you've had a bath with my son!"

She blushed bright red and hurried out, however she wasn't about to be beaten and when she came back in she looked Bob straight in the eye and said, "You know when you won the Grand National?"

"Yes," Bob said with a bit of a preening look to him.

"I wasn't even born!"

That was definitely Bob put in his place and we have reminded him of it on several occasions."

I do remember that night. Just goes to show what a very small world it is sometimes!

"Even on his wedding reception to Dee he played up. We'd left the venue and had stopped to have a drink at Wheelers, a local pub and had only been there a few minutes when Bob sat down next to us. He said, "I thought I'd have more fun here!"

In fairness to me, we'd actually been married a week and this was just the official reception. Dee didn't even know I'd gone!

"After he won the National it was as though he became a different person, not to us of course, but from that day on it was, 'Bob Champion Cancer Survivor'. It's as though that title has been tacked on to the end of his name. The cancer is a part of who he is but isn't him.

I hope that people understand just how good he is to people who have cancer and who are really unwell. We had a friend who was terminally ill and she asked if we could get her a copy of Bob's book. When I asked him if he could send us one to post to her he said no, asked us where she was being treated and went off to see her with a signed copy. He spent a few hours with her chatting and telling her stories. She died a few weeks later, but had said that his visit meant so much to her."

I do love Sally. I call her 'Mum' and she's absolutely brilliant.

Every morning I'm grateful to wake up. I think anyone who has been as close to death as I have is likely to feel the same way. It's a realisation that another day is a gift to be used and not wasted. The emotions of it all are complicated, of course they are, but I do wholeheartedly agree with what Ed Chamberlain said.

Like him, I carry an immense amount of guilt that I survived when so many didn't. That is why I push myself so hard and intend to carry on for as long as I possibly can.

The Final Furlong

I was delighted to have been invited to take part in the BBC documentary programme, The Real Marigold Hotel in September 2017. It will be going to air at roughly the same time this book comes out, but for several months I had to keep quiet about it as the producers like the identity of the celebrities' kept secret until closer to the launch.

This marked my first TV appearance in many years and I was quite nervous. You're filmed for up to fifteen hours a day and they have three film crews along to capture every moment. At the time of writing I have no idea how I'll feel seeing myself on TV after so many years, I hope that it's my natural charm that comes across and not the grumpy man easily irritated! I think I was just my natural self, although I was under strict instructions from both Janette and Lucy that I behave and not show myself up! I have no idea what they were talking about.

If you haven't seen the programme, the format is quite simple; they take eight 'celebrity' pensioners and put them in a hotel in India with a small weekly 'pension' and see if they would like to actually retire and live out there. The concept of it came about after the release of the movie, 'The Best Exotic Marigold Hotel' which starred a great collection of British actors, including Dame Judi Dench and Dame Maggie Smith. The film follows a group of

British retirees who decide to outsource their retirement to less expensive and seemingly exotic India. Some clever person came up with the idea of trying it out for real with a collection of older celebrities.

I was incredibly worried to see who I would be spending four weeks filming with. Again it was kept very hush-hush before filming commenced. I actually met one of the camera men at a horse show the day before I was due to fly out and I asked him if he'd tell me who was going. Well, I can certainly confirm that the beeb know how to pick their teams as he was very tight lipped and wouldn't say a word.

The week prior to flying out I was travelling here there and everywhere. I'd spent two days with my publisher prepping this book and visiting the Trust in Norwich, then I was off on a two day golf and speaking gig in Derby. The night before I was due to fly out I was giving an after-dinner speech and then I drove back home to Newmarket. I arrived home at 2am and the car picked me up at 2.30am to take me to Heathrow. Thankfully Janette had packed everything ready for me and being as organised as she is I knew I didn't have to worry too much. I was determined to be smartly dressed whilst over there, perhaps reminiscent of an old colonial Englishman.

As I arrived at Heathrow I was quite anxious, I'd arrived first and I was probably showing signs of impatience as I don't like waiting for anything. They did offer me a list of who was travelling with me at that point, but I declined. I figured I'd waited this long I might as well get the full surprise effect.

My fellow travellers, in no particular order were Peter Dean who'd played Pete Beale in EastEnders, The Krankies, Janette and Ian (my goodness they were to take India by storm), Syd Little, and Stanley Johnson, Boris's Dad. I knew straight away that Syd and I would get on and throughout the trip we had a great deal of fun, but I'll tell you more about that later. Susan George, Selena Scott and Stephanie Beacham were our female companions. It was interesting as I'd never met any of them before and we were filmed introducing ourselves.

After that it was off though customs to departures where we rested until our flight was called. The crew wanted to keep us from chatting at that point as they were looking to film us getting to know one another so we really weren't encouraged to mingle. We were all tired anyway so that wasn't too much of an issue. We headed off and I watched movies mostly for the journey out. Arriving into India, we stayed in Mumbai the first night and from that point on we were filmed constantly. It was our first taste of what the next few weeks were going to be like. Next day we flew to Udaipur and travelled to the private hotel. It was very, very nice and run by such lovely people. In fact from the hotel you could see where the Bond movie, Octopussy, had been filmed.

Now… here I was in India and at the age I am, you would probably have thought I had tried their national dish many, many times. But no. I had my very first curry that evening.

I'm sorry to say, my immediate thought was, 'Ughh, I hate this' and I'm even more afraid to tell you that my opinion didn't change for the whole trip. I'm not a fan of spicy food, so I knew I was going to be in for a rough time. I mean, who'd have thought that being in India we would have curry every night! There were also a lot of vegetables and I'm not fond of those either. I did get used to the naan bread though. Before too long everyone on set knew that I didn't like curries, no matter how much I tried to put on a brave face for the cameras and the crew often took delight in winding me up. I don't think I'll ever have another curry in my life. My treat when we weren't filming was to go to the restaurant and have cheese and mushrooms on toast. That was a real pleasure. I did drink more Coca-Cola than was good for me and the odd glass of wine. The desserts were nice though and I've already mentioned my sweet tooth so I wasn't going to starve.

To keep things moving along, the crew would introduce themes for us to talk about and it worked quite well, although we were probably a bit cheekier off camera as I know we wouldn't have wanted to say anything that would have caused offence. I'd have been in trouble at home if I had!

I did really enjoy it though, regardless of the curry sagas. I had a great time with everyone. Syd Little was a lot of fun and we did get up to a few cheeky moments, he always made me laugh. Stanley, Boris's Dad, is a clever, clever man, who I admired a great deal. He's as eccentrically dressed as his son, but it seemed there wasn't anything he didn't know about. I did feel for him though as he was constantly being contacted by the media about Boris. I asked him if he thought his boy would make a good Prime Minister and he said, "Yes, of course. He has a very clever mind and some brilliant ideas. It's just a shame that in parliament your best friends would stab you in the back if it meant they'd get on better and it's quite a lonely life."

Selena was a top class journalist and it showed. I know she never meant to do it, but you often felt that when she spoke to you, you were being interviewed. I imagine it is a difficult habit to get out of, but she totally stunned me when she revealed that not only had we attended the same school, but that her form tutor had been good old Mr McKenzie! What a very small world! We spent quite the time reminiscing about him. I think Selena must have been very, very bright for our school and she was Head Girl.

Susan George and I had a lot in common as she has a stud farm that breeds Arabian horses, so we talked a lot about that. It's not surprising that we would also discuss the loss of her husband, Simon MacCorkindale, from cancer. His death hit her hard and she still misses him. She was a lovely person, but my goodness me what a top professional she was, even if she was annoyed or upset with something, once the cameras were rolling, you could never have told. I wish I could have done that! It must be marvellous to switch off your feelings and simply 'be' I think most people can tell if I'm not happy.

The queen of the group was Stephanie. She certainly had that star-presence. I'll be honest, I thought she and I would clash, but far from it. In actual fact, I really liked her and I admired her way of gently persuading the hotel staff into fulfilling her every need. She would always be last to arrive so that she had the best entrance and she always got her own way, but not in a mean or nasty sense. She was lovely once she relaxed and all in all we got on fabulously. Like Susan, she could flick the professional switch and you couldn't tell her emotions. Stephanie could sweep in to a room as though she was still in Dynasty. Sad to say, I'd just bumble through the door.

The person that amazed me the most though, was Janette of the Krankies. She has an utterly stunning personality and wherever she went children followed her. It was like watching the Pied Piper. They adored her and she was always so much fun and full of life. To be fair, I think she stole the show, but you'll have to let me know when you watch it. Ian was her perfect straight man and they were A1 together, a true partnership in all senses.

You know one thing I found, was that everyone we met was always cheerful. They might not have had a great deal of material goods, but they were constantly laughing and they made the most of what they had. They were all so friendly.

A few days into the trip we were invited to try some yoga and afterwards none of us could walk! I think they'd neglected to mention that some of us were old crocs, although I did get some exercises that were supposed to help. Doing them out in the warm climate of India certainly did, but in cold wet England I haven't even tried. I may get around to them but the yoga thing was a tough workout and a hard ninety minutes.

To make up for nearly wrecking us, we were invited to visit the Amber Fort, near Jaipur. Wow, what a place. How they built it I'll never know and I don't think we could replicate it today. Did you know that in times of attack they could hold 1,000 horses there and had enough food for a month's siege? Having their own well in the castle grounds meant their water couldn't be contaminated either. I'll admit to being in awe and totally fascinated by the place. As Pete is a practising Buddhist he was also fascinated by the architecture of the places of worship and he shared some truly beautiful insights. It must be a calm and tranquil way for the soul. He also had quite a few on-set stories from EastEnders that were perhaps not so good on the soul.

I already knew that I'd be asked to play some polo whilst out there, so it was no surprise, but if you haven't seen it yet, you may need to lower your expectations. I say play, but I mean we knocked some balls about with the professionals. I really don't ride anymore so it was a bit of a shock to my old muscles, but you never lose the skills, although I think Howard and Derek may comment adversely on my riding style. It was fun to be back in the saddle and the gentle polo introduction was a good thing as they had future riding planned towards the end of the four weeks.

In Jodhpur we attended an official function and I was gifted a traditional headpiece. I think it really suited me, but the responses I've had from those who've seen the pictures, leads me to believe that it perhaps wasn't as flattering as I first thought. I did hear one reference to Carmen Miranda, but I ignored it.

Syd, me, Ian and Janette had become fed up with curries, so one night we decided that we were going to cook. Now Syd Little can cook as he owned a restaurant and I'd done Ready-Steady-Cook, where you will remember I'd been 'robbed' of victory, so we figured, 'how hard could it be?' We went off to the local market and realised, 'quite hard' was the answer. We had a dreadful time trying to buy what we needed and in the end I said, "Leave it to me."

I approached a local lady and asked her to help us out. Fortunately for us she did, including not over-paying and we managed to get everything we needed at the right prices, except meat. Of course we couldn't have beef as that's sacred, so we'd decided on lamb. We got taken to a back street butchers where I kept asking for lamb and the guys kept pointing out cuts to me that looked nothing like any lamb I'd ever seen. After a lot of hand gestures and lots more wrangling, they took us out the back to show us the 'lamb' which turned out to be a goat! We decided to go for chicken instead and they asked us to pick the ones we wanted, which we did. There and then they chopped off their heads and put them into a machine that plucked them whilst still flapping. Now, having my Dad knackering I've seen some things, but this was a bit much even for me! We went back and cooked a lovely meal and one I was actually able to eat.

I did have a few moments of 'Deli Belly' which I of course put down to all the curry. We'd been taken to see the doctor over there a few times, to compare UK to Indian medical treatments. He was a strange little man and if I'm honest I thought he was a quack! My back had been playing up and so he suggested that the cause was my body adsorbing toxins and not flushing them out correctly. His remedy? An enema. Now as you'll already have read, I'm no stranger to these, or so I thought. I was expecting a small pill but what came out was a steel pipe, brown bag and a ten-inch long tube. Everything looked like it was dated from the 1800's! I had the sudden realisation that an enema was something entirely different in India. Whilst he was inserting it, I clearly remember saying 'I won't ever be gay' but I doubt they'll show that bit! I'd love to tell you that it worked and that my back pain eased, but it didn't and the 'Deli Belly' came back with a vengeance! The rest of the crew thought it was highly amusing, but I think I'll stick to traditional pain relief from now on.

We had a fascinating insight into Indian society when we attended a Fiesta in Ahmedabad. To get there we needed to go on an overnight train, and I was pleased to hear we were travelling first class. Ha! I love travelling to new places and one thing that you can rely on is that terms like first class are always relative. Imagine mid-summer on an overly crammed slow train heading to the seaside in Britain and then times the heat and the crowding by ten! We were lucky enough to have bunks, so I had Stanley above me and we had a married couple in the bunk opposite. The wife was heavily, and I mean heavily, pregnant so I prayed that she didn't go into labour overnight, can you imagine me, the midwife?

The toilet... Well... that was an intriguing arrangement. It was basically just a hole in the floor and what with the heat, the smell was worse than anything I'd ever known in my life and I've worked on farms. I don't even want to imagine what it was like for those poor souls travelling in what I can only describe as 'cattle class'. They had no windows, just bars on the side and nowhere to sleep. It must have been hell for them. Though, different as they were, the trains did run precisely on time and weren't stopped by leaves on the line.

We arrived for the Fiesta, and found that we would be staying in a lovely modern hotel, but being a 'dry state' it meant we were back to drinking coke.

We were given a teacher as we needed to learn how to dance and if final proof was needed that 'Strictly' is not for me, then this was it. I think I managed to stumble around in a circle then it was off to find outfits for the next day. This was actually harder than it sounds as the Indians tend to be a lot smaller of build than us tubby English folk. But we found some lovely outfits and were looking forward to the next day.

We were collected by our dance teacher and escorted to the event. I thought it would be like an English summer fete but in fact there were thousands of people there, all brightly dressed and dancing in circles. What a stunning festival and it will stay with me always. I think it might even have been a local pick-up point for the younger ones as it was a chance to get away from the ever observant parents.

The next day we went back to the 'Marigold' and I noticed that by now we had started to call it home. I realised that we probably needed to be headed back to England soon, although there was time for one last trip.

Myself, Susan and Selena were given the opportunity for an eight hour horse trek, obviously I was to be first choice for this activity although I didn't look the professional when my horse stumbled on uneven ground and went down! Luckily he didn't go all the way down and I managed to keep some dignity. We eventually arrived at what looked like a Roman war camp with square tents! Each one was modestly equipped with a bed with a single sheet. It got very cold in the night and I mean it was freezing. I was chilled to the bone and eventually got up at 4am to put my clothes back on, but they were soaking wet with condensation. I hadn't thought of that. Neither had Susan as I saw her walking around the camp a few minutes later in exactly the same damp, frozen state as myself! It took me at least an hour and a half to get warm. The toilet, well, you've never seen anything like it. It made the one on the train seem quite classy. For this one you had to practically be a gymnast to get in it as it was so high up and on wheels. It was just that, a tin shed on wheels up in the air. A shower meant walking down to the river and getting a bucket of water, carrying it back to the tin shed and pouring it over your head. You could have saved yourself the trip by washing in the river, but you'd have likely been eaten! I'm afraid to say that none of us showered until we were in the safety of our hotel rooms. Probably just as well it isn't surround smell television.

We did have a good meal up there though and no, it wasn't curry!

There was only one thing that frustrated me during the whole time I was there and that was the slight disorganisation. I realise, given that you have read this far through my book, that this revelation may shock you, but... I'm not a patient man. So when someone says we're leaving at 9am I expect to leave at 9am and not be standing around waiting whilst they load the vehicles at 9am. That's not what race time means to me. If it says the 3.45 at Ascot, it means we're running at 3.45, not still in the parade ring. I did bite my tongue, a lot, but that was the only niggle I had.

I'm really glad that I did it and I thoroughly enjoyed my time in India. It is an exceptional country. As I'm writing this 'I'm a Celebrity Get Me Out of Here' is being aired and it's been a pleasure to watch Stanley in the jungle. I knew that he would do well and would give it his very best, but I wasn't at all surprised to see Toff winning as she is as bright as a button!

I'm looking forward to more shows coming up and you may end up seeing more of me than you expected, but I won't give anything away just yet.

I also recently received another formal letter inviting me to join a rather exclusive club, however this time it's for naughty school. I know, I know, I should have been driving at 30mph but in my defence having caught an 80-year-old lady that day too, I think the community officers' machines must have needed calibrating. I'm not making light of the need to drive carefully and I feel angrier at myself for having made such a stupid mistake. I was due to attend in November 2017 but was actually sick on the day and they sent me home. That never happened at my real school but the Driving School is obviously more lenient. I shall go back and take my punishment.

Thinking ahead as I have to do, I have decided to donate my brain to research. Seriously. Not just me either. The Jockey Club asked a number of us as part of the investigation into impact sport and the effects of concussion. So far the results of the tests show that I don't have 100% feeling in my hands and feet and that although the memory test showed I wasn't too bad, I wasn't happy with my results. I know that there must be repercussions to the amount of times we jockeys hit our heads. The long-term results of concussion are seriously damaging, but we really didn't have a clue back in the day. I mean, I was thirty-years old before I ever wore a helmet to ride out. The first helmets we wore in races were very flimsy, like they were made from cardboard, offered no protection and were only worn to keep our colour caps on!

Thinking of those days, I am often asked if I miss riding. The truth is, yes, but I only miss riding as a proper jockey. I don't ride for personal pleasure anymore, but that's ok, because if I can't ride the way I used to it's just not the same. I am and have always been an all or nothing man. I do occasionally ride for the Trust and of course will continue to do that, but it will take the lure of cowboys for me to consider riding seriously again.

φ

As I look back on my life and go through the pages of this book, I've realised how so many people that were close to me, or who have helped me through the worst times of my life, have now passed away. I was especially reminded of someone I cared a great deal about.

I met Shona Matheson at a race meeting back in the seventies and I thought that she was lovely inside and out. Her parents were very wealthy and I always thought that she was way too good for me, you know? Well I allowed things to drift and she went off to America and married a lovely man. I often saw her mother at the races and she would tell me how much Shona had cared for me and how she thought I'd have been good for her daughter! I'm sure everyone has someone in their life that they wonder about. You know, like a 'were they the one that got away' type of thing. Maybe Shona was mine, but things happen for a reason and I know she was truly happy with her life as I am now with mine. She and I remained firm friends and I'd stop by to visit her and her family. I received a call a couple of years ago from her daughter to tell me she'd passed away, from cancer no less. I never knew. It seems that those I am closest to are destined to be affected by this disease. They say one in three, but for me those statistics don't seem to measure up.

Another person I've been thinking a lot about whilst writing this is Josh Gifford, my Guv'nor. He played such a huge part in my life that it's no surprise that his death should have hurt me. He'd been having heart problems and he'd been ill for a little while before he passed away in February 2012. I'd seen him a few times in the month before as I'd pop in to see him when I was down there. Then I received the call a few hours after he died. I was absolutely gutted. He was a great man and I was really upset. I went to his memorial at Chichester Cathedral and he was so popular that it was standing room only. The press reported more than 800 people attended. It was a fitting testimony to and a mark of, the man. It's nice nowadays when I see Tina, Nick and Althea and it's good to keep that connection.

Josh gave me such good advice throughout my time with him, none better than when he said, "When you pull up, think about the race, because your first impression will always be the right one."

That's advice I've used not only in racing but in all aspects of my life and it has never steered me wrong. Never a man for a lot of compliments, he was a real professional and perhaps harder to ride for when you were doing well as he liked to keep you grounded, but if you were having a bad run he'd always pick you up. A 'well done' from Josh Gifford was all you ever needed. I think that of all the people I ever knew, he had the biggest influence on my life. Mind you, the words of Toby Balding have also stayed with me. In my first few days with him he said, "Bob, two things you need to know in life, no two horses will ever act the same way and women ain't people." He was certainly right… Well, about the horses!

Despite the passing of so many, I am still incredibly lucky and especially because my two best friends, Howard and Derek Thompson are still around. Yorkshire has always been and I'm sure always will be where I consider home. Going back there and staying with Howard is a real delight. I'm so pleased that he and Tina are involved in racehorses and although I maintain they're a great way to get poor quick, they're loving their stables. I do enjoy winding Howard up when he goes to the horse sales but it's all good fun. When he, Derek and I get together we're just like little boys again and some things will never change. Their Mum laughs at us and I'm so fortunate to have them as my family. Like all best mates we banter and tease and cajole and rarely, like most men our age, do we say what we feel. I'm not about to start now. But they know. As do I.

It is such a pleasure to be surrounded by good friends and I do better than most, I know. I stay with Jonathan Powell and his wife Charlotte quite often and we spend time at the races. Ian Watkinson lives close by, so we often nip out for a drink in the evening. We're a pair of rascals and love reminiscing. Although Ian is far, far worse than me!

As I consider though, how many old friends are gone, it would seem that I am getting closer to facing my own mortality again, although this time there is no cure for simply getting old. Don't get me wrong, I have no desire to ship off yet. Both Mum and Dad were a good age when they died and I fully expect to be the same, so I am still making plans for what to do with the great expanse of years I have left to me.

I'm very tempted to take myself off and find a holiday where I can ride the range like a fully-fledged cowboy. It has long been a dream of mine and in fact in 2008, once I knew Janette had recovered from her cancer, I went off to Australia to go outback riding. Wow what an experience! I flew to Melbourne and got a bus out to Geelong, incidentally where Prince Charles went to school, some two hours away. Then I got a taxi to take me to the hut where I spent the evening boarding with ten others. They were from a variety of walks of life and were all very friendly. I don't know what made me do it but I decided to play down my riding ability and certainly didn't mention I'd been a professional jockey. I think they looked at me and my age and decided on day one to put me on a dobbin! It wasn't moving and after I gave it a bit of dig it still wasn't going anywhere fast. Half a day in and the staff noted that I had a good riding style and put me on a much better horse, it was lovely in fact. As was the countryside we were travelling through. What a magnificent view of plains and bush and gently rising foothills, with a backdrop of higher peaks.

After a while we started going up into the mountains and one day we were riding along a ledge that was no wider than the horse. We were literally hundreds of feet up with a sheer drop next to us and I'm riding along thinking, 'I don't like this!' I remember thinking that when they fall off a ledge in a movie there's always a tree to grab onto, so I'm looking for these imaginary trees! Of course there weren't any so I had to content myself in knowing that the horse wouldn't want to slip and die and I didn't want to die, so I best just let it do what it wanted to. We must have been climbing this ledge for an hour and I know I had a huge sense of relief when we got to the top. The smell of eucalyptus was incredible, it was all so fresh. We camped out that night and it gets cold up there, but what a sky. After this we wound our way back down and I was able to ride the horse along a riverbed. They didn't tell us that the water dropped from two feet to 250 feet deep, so I galloped straight in and the next thing I'm sat in water and the horse is swimming. The horse didn't mind and I just went with it. We camped out again that night and the next day, as the trek came to an end there was a hill with a good three furlong straight rising up it. The staff said that they always liked a race here and I thought I might just come into my own. I figured having not raced before they'd charge off and most likely not make it. I'd have a steady start, give the horse a breather, which they wouldn't and then of course I'd pass them, which I did. They all looked at me strangely and said, "It looks like you've ridden before." So I decided to come clean.

I'd do it again or like I say, do one which had the opportunity to round up cattle and that would see me very happy.

I was asked recently if I could go back in time and choose, would I suffer the cancer and have the life I've had, or choose not to have it at all. Without question I would choose not to have it. After all, you never know how your life is going to go and I may still have achieved all that I have today, maybe more. But of course you can't go back. You play the hand you are dealt and despite any hardship, I've been incredibly fortunate.

It's strange to think that I had over 500 winners in my career as a jockey, yet most only remember me as winning one race, but given which one it was, I guess that's not so bad.

My ambition as a boy was to ride in the Grand National, my ambition whilst going through chemo was to win the Grand National, so what is my ambition now? For me it's simple, I want to see a major breakthrough for the cancer trust and I know, as sure as I knew I'd ride Aldaniti and win, that we will see one.

Now, that paragraph above was meant to bring this chapter to a close. I was almost finished with the whole book. All I had left to do was to round it off with a brief thought or two in a short end piece called 'The Chair' and of course, select the photographs that would appear throughout. To do that last thing, I packed up boxes and boxes of photos that I had collected over the years, along with all the cuttings and diaries from the Cancer Trust Charity events and would, at the start of 2018, go and see my publisher, Taryn, to choose the final images.

First though, following a family Christmas, I would attend the Liverpool International Horse Show. During the three-day extravaganza they were playing host to the Shetland ponies Grand National and the Cancer Trust was once again happy to be involved with them. Normally these shows are so much fun and the Shetland events are so vibrant and fresh it's difficult to know who gets more enjoyment out of them, the ponies or the kids. I do love attending them, however this year I had come down with that dreaded flu bug and was feeling so rough that I'd had to miss the first day. Not to be deterred though I set off early on New Year's Eve 2017 to arrive in plenty of time for that day's show. In a short break between the afternoon activities and the planned evening gala events, I returned to my hotel to get changed and freshened up. That was when I first noticed the flames beginning to appear in the carpark next to the arena. The carpark where my car was.

The small fire quickly became an inferno and all I can say is a tremendous thank you to all the emergency services who managed to ensure none of the 80 horses stabled on the ground floor, none of the pet dogs who had been inside cars and most importantly not one person, was injured. Given the eventual scale of the fire and the resultant temperatures within the structure, it was a remarkable feat that the firefighters managed. Just one more example of how outstanding our emergency services, fire, police and medical are.

I knew there wasn't a hope of any vehicles surviving, but cars can be replaced, so the following day I set off home on the train. I guess I was about halfway through the journey when I realised I'd have to ring Taryn and cancel our meeting. It was then the horrible truth dawned on me. All my photos, all my diaries, all my cuttings had still been in the boot of the car.

I'm really lucky to enjoy good friends within various media outlets, so I was interviewed about the saga a couple of times and put out an appeal asking if people could donate photos of me that they might have squirreled away.

The response from friends, family and the general public was overwhelming. I received a lot of pictures from personal collections and was reminded of events that I had forgotten. The Racing Post in Liverpool kindly opened up their archives to me and a French photographer, Jean-Pierre Montbazet, offered me the use of his incredible Grand National photos.

So, I just want to say thank you to those whose photos appear in this book and equal thanks to all of those who took the time to reach out with such generosity. Your kindness to me, as always, since those heady days of the Grand National victory in 1981, still causes me to feel so humble and grateful for the life I have been fortunate to have had.

The Chair

The biggest obstacle I ever faced on a racecourse was the fifteenth fence on the Aintree Grand National course. It's called 'The Chair'.

Combining a 6ft wide open ditch with a 5ft tall and 3ft wide fence, even landing it is tricky due to the upward sloping ground. As I've mentioned before, you don't think about it. You just ride the horse, set for it right, take an extra stride, or stand off as far as you dare, then attack it. You never consider falling off and if you were to, you just roll small, wait for the other hooves to pass you by, get up and carry on. Looking forward to the next time when you will do better. When you will clear it, land it and go on to win the race.

I look at cancer treatment and think the same. Set your mind right. Ride the treatment out. Clear the obstacles and if you falter, get up and try again. And again and again.

Yes, I did all of that and people lauded me for it. But, I shall never forget and no fellow sufferers should either, that it was the courage, resilience, unstinting happiness and positivity of a ward full of children that made me succeed. For at my lowest, my most despairing, 'give it up' moment, those children gave me the resolve and the determination to overcome any obstacle.

I can look back across all those years and be truly thankful for that child, rocking backwards and forwards on her toy horse, looking straight at me with the innocence and openness of unfiltered honesty as she asked me that one simple question:

"Are you going to die, or are you going to live?"
"I'm going to live."

With courage like they showed, you can overcome anything.
Bob Champion MBE
2018

Annex

John Francome

In preparing this book I have obviously spent a lot of time reflecting on the past and on horse racing, a sport that has been my life. I still enjoy it immensely and I thought it might be fun to profile a few of the top names in trainers and jockeys that I've had the pleasure of knowing. Some of them are contemporary with me, some are relative youngsters in my eyes, but all are people I find fascinating. As well as their notable achievements I'll add why I personally think they are the special ones of racing. I can't begin anywhere else than with the man I think was the classiest jumper of them all.

He's been described as the 'best jockey never to have won a Grand National', but John Francome MBE is, in my opinion, the best there was. Yes, I know that by statistics he's the third most successful jump jockey behind AP McCoy and Peter Scudamore, but I can choose to think differently.

I always find it interesting to see where the great horsemen and women have come from in terms of background and a lot are obviously born into horse-centric families, but this wasn't the case with John. His Dad was actually a railway fireman, but despite the lack of obvious connections with horses, John developed an interest through a love of show jumping. By the time he was sixteen he had become apprenticed to the rather formidable Fred Winter. Based down in Lambourn, he won his first race at seventeen and went on to ride a total of 1,138 winners. On his surprise, I would actually say shock, retirement at Chepstow in April 1985, he was then the most successful jump jockey in history.

After hanging up his riding boots, he was awarded the MBE in 1986 for services to racing and went on to be a trainer for eighteen months. However, with the move of racing coverage to Channel-4, John became a well-opinionated and occasionally controversial, but always polite, racing pundit. I used to love watching him and Derek on the Morning Line. It made for great television.

He continued in the role for twenty-seven years and he and Derek left at the same time when the franchise moved on. He's also an accomplished author having written more than twenty racing thrillers and two autobiographies.

John was also committed to giving something back to our game and was the president of the Injured Jockeys Fund before handing over to AP in 2016. He's now the Vice-Patron of the fund in support of Her Royal Highness the Princess Royal.

There's no question in my mind that John Francome is the best National Hunt jockey of all time. I know that his records of winners and Champion Jockey titles would get beaten later, but John oozed class in the saddle. I have never seen a better rider over an obstacle. It did help that he'd been Junior European Show Jumping Champion before he came into racing, but whether it was that or just natural ability, it was evident each time he took to the track.

Whatever he did or does, he's so professional and driven. Be it horse racing or Tiddlywinks, John would be the best at it. Add to all of that a wickedly dry sense of humour and some killer one-liners and you have a man that was always popular in the weighing room. He was mostly perfect going over obstacles and he sat well throughout a race. That sense of balance shouldn't be underestimated and John had it at his core, wrapped in style.

Vincent O'Brien

Saying that Michael Vincent O'Brien, born in County Cork, Ireland in 1917, was an Irish race horse trainer, is like saying Muhammad Ali was a kid who could fight a bit.

Understanding that he started out as a greyhound trainer, then moved to point-to-points, then National Hunt, then flat racing and finally helped establish the most influential breeding stud in racing's history, is a bit more of an insight into the man who was the 'master'.

Realising that he was voted in a Racing Post worldwide poll as the greatest influence in horse racing history, probably allows you to grasp the truth. There was never anyone, before or since, who has reached across the racing world like he did. Given my background, I find it interesting that his father was a farmer who regularly took part in fox-hunting.

In a stellar career, Vincent trained six horses to win the Epsom Derby, was twice British champion trainer, won three Grand Nationals in succession and trained the only British Triple Crown winner there has been since before the Second World War, Nijinsky.

The magnificence of that achievement alone is the mark of the man and of course, his flat racing statistics were assisted by the jockey he had in the saddle more often than not, Lester Piggott. The two shared an amazingly illustrious and long partnership. In fact when Vincent trained his last winner, at Royal Ascot in 1993, Lester was on board and their combined age that day was 133.

In tandem with the training, along with Tim Vigors and Robert Sangster, he founded the Coolmore stud and began to bring across some top American thoroughbreds to introduce back into the

English racing line. The success that the stud and its racing arm 'Ballydoyle' had and continues to have is unmatched.

To list all of Vincent's major races would take up an awful lot of space, but suffice to say that with 16 English Classics, 27 Irish Classics, three Prix de L'arc de Triomphes, three Champion Hurdles, three Grand Nationals and four Cheltenham Gold Cups, he had a record that whilst some may surpass bits of it, it's unlikely anyone will match it all.

On all the occasions I ever met him he was pleasant, quiet and reserved. A proper gentleman who carried the mantle of genius easily.

Jonjo O'Neill

"Jonjo" O'Neill was born in 1952 and is another great horseman to come from County Cork, Ireland. Perhaps they have a factory down there? His boyhood ambition was to become a jockey and after leaving school he began an apprenticeship with Michael Connolly. In 1970 he rode his first winner and three years later, Jonjo moved to be based in the north of England, From then on his career went from strength to strength.

In 1977/78, he broke the record for most winners in a season with a total of 149, beating the previous record, held by former champion Ron Barry, by twenty-four. The following season, he claimed the Jockeys' Championship for a second successive time. John Francome commented that to win two Jockeys' titles whilst based in the far north of England was 'the equivalent of winning five Olympic Gold Medals' and it's true. That was a tremendous achievement.

During his career, Jonjo was associated with many fine horses, including Alverton, on which he won the first of his two Cheltenham Gold Cups, just ahead of Royal Mail in second and me on Aldaniti in third. Jonjo also rode the marvellous Night Nurse and Sea Pigeon, although it's arguably his second Gold Cup winning mount, the mare Dawn Run, that most will remember. She became the only horse to complete the double of winning the Champion Hurdle and the Gold Cup at the Cheltenham Festival, both times with Jonjo on board.

Overall he won a staggering 900 races as a jockey and then made the transition to trainer almost seamlessly. Well, apart from being diagnosed with cancer. I could hardly believe it. After fighting his own battle against the disease, during which time he still came out to support the Bob Champion Trust, he made it through and recovered fully.

He has since gone on to establish himself as one of the most successful race horse trainers of the modern era and since moving to his stables up at Jackdaws Castle in the heart of the Cotswolds, he continues to be outstanding. With more than 2,000 winners trained he has a big race record that is phenomenal, including a remarkable twenty-six Cheltenham Festival winners including a Gold Cup with Synchronicity and of course, he brought Don't Push It to Grand National victory, thereby giving AP McCoy his only National win.

Jonjo was fortunate that he was light and could ride on the flat as well as over jumps, but he was immensely strong. A man gifted with an incredible amount of charisma he was and continues to be a fun and all-round nice bloke. When he was diagnosed with cancer, I found all my old fears and anger at that disease coming back to mind, but it was so good that he battled his way through it.

I know also that as a mark of how peculiar our sport can be, Jonjo's record in the Grand National speaks volumes. In the seven attempts he rode in the race, this jockey with unerring abilities and a terrifically competitive, yet fair, nature never got further than the Canal Turn second time round. It goes to show how much the planets have to line up for success in that particular race.

Peter Scudamore

Peter Scudamore MBE, known by all of us jockeys as Scu', was Champion Jockey eight times, including one title shared with John Francome. Another member of the '1,000 winner's club' with 1,678, he came from great racing stock, with his father, Michael winning the National on Oxo in 1959 and the Gold Cup on Linwell in 1957.

At the age of twenty, Scu' was relatively late starting out in his first competitive race, but over the next fifteen years he went on to become statistically the second greatest National Hunt jockey of all time. Although both his total winners and winners in one season records have been surpassed now, his achievements still boggle the mind.

He rode thirteen Cheltenham Festival winners including two Champion Hurdles and a Queen Mother Champion Chase. Away from Prestbury Park he won two Hennessy Gold Cups, a Mackeson Gold Cup, four Welsh Nationals and two Scottish Nationals, although in all his attempts he never managed to secure a Grand National. Yet again another pointer to how much luck and good fortune is needed for that race.

He had some terrific seasons with Martin Pipe and I always thought his most outstanding ability was that he was a magnificent judge of pace. He seemed to instinctively know when to pick up the ride and drive home. That and his almost encyclopaedic knowledge of the form book. What he didn't know about the other horses in a race wasn't worth knowing. That is such an important aspect of being a jockey that is often overlooked. You need to know who the other horses are, what their form is, what they have done and might do. Knowing that helps you judge when to attack in the closing stages. Scu' did that so well and it's great now to see both his sons forging out their own brilliant racing careers.

Fred Winter

Fred Winter CBE was born in 1926 and his exploits might be fading in the popular consciousness of most of today's young race goers, but Fred dominated racing when I was growing up and through to the 1980s.

First as a jockey, and then as a trainer, he was one of only two people in the post-war era to be both Champion Jockey and Champion Trainer. He was also one of only three men to ride and later train a Grand National winner and unique in his winning of the Grand National, the Champion Hurdle and the Gold Cup as both a trainer and a jockey.

Champion Jockey four times and Champion Trainer eight, he was the only person I knew in our game that was never argued with. Or if he was, you weren't going to be riding for him for long.

He was a flat jockey at first, but then after serving in the Parachute Regiment during World War II, he came home and started riding over jumps. He teamed up with Captain Ryan Price and over the next two decades he notched up 923 winners including the Champion Hurdle three times, the Triumph Hurdle twice and the Grand National, with Kilmore, in 1962. He retired from riding in 1964 and became the first jockey to be awarded the CBE for his services to racing.

This outstanding jockey then went on to make the transition to be an outstanding trainer with a great affinity for his horses. His continued success and his intimate knowledge of the game meant that he would always benefit from having the top jockeys riding for him, but my goodness me, what he said went. You always did as you were told when Fred gave you an instruction, but I reckon his bark was worse than his bite. I just decided never to test my theory.

John Francome was a stable lad for him and later a jockey, but one day early on in his career at the stables, John took a car to the wrong location and had to ring his Guv'nor to explain what had happened.

"I apologised to him and said I'd be on my way. The boss just growled back at me, 'That's all right, son; it's not your fault, it's my fault. You're so bloody stupid, I should have put up a blackboard and written your instructions on it.'"

Grumpy or gruff, plain spoken or blunt, it didn't matter because the man could train horses, which is strange given that he never really wanted to in the first place. He had only gotten into it after he'd been turned down in his wish to become a starter.

But a record of Grand Nationals, Gold Cups, Champion Hurdles, the King George VI Chase and the Two Mile Champion Chase are unequivocal in testimony to his talents.

Sadly he was to suffer two strokes in his retirement years, but I'd see him around and about at events and functions and his resolve was undiminished.

Richard Dunwoody

Belfast born Richard Dunwoody MBE, is the only jockey of his generation to win the Grand National, the Gold Cup and the Champion Hurdle and thereby complete the National Hunt's 'Big Three'. He also had four victories in the King George VI Chase, on two of the greatest steeplechasers in National Hunt history, winning in 1989 and 1990 on Desert Orchid and again in 1995 and 1996 on One Man. When I've spoken to him in the past he's said that he considered that his best rides and wins were on the great Desert Orchid and having seen them in full flight, I can't argue. Richard had seven wins on him, including the Irish Grand National.

He won the Aintree Grand National twice. First in 1986 on West Tip and then again on Miinnehoma in 1994 and was Champion Jockey three times between 1993 and 1995. Joining the illustrious ranks of the '1,000 winner's club' he was awarded the MBE for services to his sport in 1993. Sadly, despite continued success, he was forced to take early retirement on the advice of doctors because of advancing arthritis that threatened potentially serious neck damage.

Since retiring in 1999, he has been a terrific patron for charities and has raised tens of thousands of pounds for various causes. He's also undertaken expeditions to both the Arctic and Antarctic. In 2003 he competed in the inaugural Polar Race and in 2008 he completed an unsupported expedition to the South Pole, travelling around 700miles on skis. In 2017, to raise funds for Sarcoma UK, he walked the length of Japan's three largest islands covering over 2000miles in 101 days.

As well as all of that, he is also a great photographer and in 2011 he signed up to a nine month intensive photojournalism course at the Spéos Photographic Institute in Paris.

In my opinion Richard is one of the most dedicated professionals I've ever met. He would be meticulous in his preparation and knew the course and the horse in a way that was somehow a cut above the rest. He was definitely the man you wanted for the big races.

I also ponder quirks like how Richard, who was Champion Jockey in the three years immediately before AP's twenty years of dominance began, was born less than forty miles away from the great McCoy. How is it that such a small place like Northern Ireland can gift the world such exceptional talents?

Don Cantillon

Now there is a chance that if you are not really into your racing, you may have encountered the name above and said, "Who?" But within racing circles Don is a trainer that when he speaks about a horse, or indeed runs a horse, people tend to sit up, take notice and listen.

He operates a small training operation in Newmarket and has a select string of both flat and National Hunt horses, but he has excelled in buying cheap and bringing on some amazing talents. This in an industry where the fairy-tale of taking a cast aside thoroughbred in a field and turning it into a Derby or a Grand National winner is much rarer than in the past and it wasn't that prevalent back then.

He also uses a wide variety of training methods and isn't scared to swap them up if needed, but whatever he does, works. I remember back in 2003, he bought a horse called That Look for about £1,000. By 2010 when he retired it, the horse had run fourteen times on the flat and twelve times over jumps. Winning a total of eight times, placing a further five that gelding brought in nearly £30,000 in prize money for its owner Mr Orbell. That type of an eye and the ability to prepare them correctly is a rare talent.

Whenever Don lays one out it isn't often it gets beat and I am firmly of the opinion that if he wanted more horses he could have more winners. He's one of the unsung talents in the game and a funny and amicable personality to boot.

ANNEX

Adrian Maguire

Beginning out in Irish pony racing at the age of nine, Adrian Maguire, who was born in 1971 in County Meath, Ireland, has been described as the greatest jump jockey never to win the Champion Jockey title.

With 1,024 race winners in the UK, his first winner in England came at the Cheltenham Festival in 1991. Imagine that. It's the equivalent of your first goal scored being the winning strike in the World Cup, or the first mountain you climb being Everest. Needless to say, Adrian's win on Omerta flung him into the spotlight of publicity. I've known jockeys go their whole career and not win at Cheltenham and here was this slip of a young man sauntering over from Ireland and winning in his first Festival. The predictions were that he could go on to be a great. I had to agree because he reminded me so much, through the style of him, of a young Jonjo O'Neill.

I read an article by Richard Edmondson that made me laugh, when he wrote, "Maguire conveyed to his mounts… that he was going over the other side of a fence and they could join him if they cared. They usually did."

Certainly with his victory in the Cheltenham Gold Cup the following year, on the tremendous Cool Ground, it looked a certainty that he would be Champion Jockey sooner rather than later, but despite being runner-up for the championship in the 1993/94 season it wasn't to be.

However, he amassed a magnificent collection of big race wins, including the Irish and Scottish Grand Nationals, the Hennessy Gold Cup, the King George VI Chase, a Triumph Hurdle, a Queen Mother Champion Chase and a Whitbread Gold Cup. Add a third place in the Grand National on Moorcroft Boy in 1994 and Adrian was a great rider for the big events. He also notably won the first five winners on a six-race card at Plumpton in 1994, before pulling up his final ride of the day. This feat of five winners was to be repeated on the Racing Post Chase Day at Kempton in 1997. I once rode four in one day and it is a tremendous effort to do it. To take five out and to do it twice is no mean feat.

Sadly though he had a lot of major injuries and bad falls and finally they all began to take a toll. In March 2002, aged just thirty-one, he fell at Warwick, breaking his neck and narrowly avoiding paralysis.

Retiring to become a trainer, he is now based in Lombard-stown, County Cork.

I always liked young Adrian, who for some reason that I don't know, got the nickname of 'The Housewives' Choice'. He was a great shape for a jockey and very strong for his size. Like I said, he reminded me of Jonjo. I think if you wanted to point out a 'complete jockey' then you wouldn't go far wrong with Adrian. He's also a thoroughly great guy with it and I was so relieved when he recovered from what we all worried was going to be a devastating injury.

AP McCoy

AP, or to give him his well-deserved proper title, Sir Anthony Peter McCoy, OBE, is the Northern Irishman who, by a massive margin, is the most successful National Hunt jockey of all time. He was apprenticed to Jim Bolger at his Coolcullen stables and I think that is where his winning mindset came from, but he had so much more in his tool bag. That he was driven and a great jockey is not up for debate, but more than that, I always felt that he could get wins on horses that no one else in the world would have got. He seemed to be able to have a sixth-sense for when to push on and when to hold back.

I always think that genius is an overused word, but when I think of Henry Cecil, Vincent O'Brien, Aidan O'Brien, Lester Piggott and AP McCoy, it's easy to use it. When it comes to being a jockey, to be called a genius I believe you need to have a collection of skills. Of course you have to be a horseman and by that I mean you need to have an intuitive relationship with each ride, know what they feel and how they can be coaxed and cajoled to give their best. Added to that, is the need to be a good judge of pace, to understand how the rest of the field is travelling, to know the form book so you know the opposition, know where the winning post is, which in simple terms means be aware of the whole race around you and know when to press for the win. Finally, you need to be aware of yourself, fit and capable and able to communicate your will through to the horse. To have all of that at the highest of levels, consistently and on tap at your beck and call, is what I think makes a genius of a jockey.

AP's statistics make for amazing reading. He was born in 1974 and even for a National Hunt jockey, at 5ft 10inches he's a tall fellow. He got his first winner when he was seventeen, riding the Jim Bolger trained Legal Steps, in a flat race at Thurles racecourse in Ireland on the 26th March 1992. Twenty-three years later on the 9th September 2015, he rode his 4,358th winner at the age of forty-one. It was a brief, one-off return to the track after officially retiring the previous April and was a fitting way to bow out.

He won his first Champion Jockey at the end of his first professional season in 95/96 and wouldn't relinquish the title until twenty years later, winning his last championship in the season of his retirement. Even before turning full professional he had won the Conditional Jump Jockeys Title with a record 74 winners under Toby Balding, my old Guv'nor. He's also received twenty 'Lesters', the racing industry's annual awards.

With regard to big race wins, well he's won almost everything there is to win. A staggering thirty-one Cheltenham Festival successes included two Gold Cups, three Champion Hurdles and a Queen Mother Champion Chase. Away from the Festival he won five Christmas Hurdles, two World Series Hurdles, a King George VI Chase and a complete set of Nationals including the Irish, Scottish, Welsh, Midland and, at his fifteenth attempt, the Aintree Grand National in 2010 on Jonjo's Don't Push It.

He was named BBC Sports Personality of the Year in 2010, becoming the first jockey to win the award. He was also awarded Sportsperson of the Year in 2010 by the Sports Journalists' Association and was the RTÉ Sports Person of the Year in 2013. In 2016 he was knighted in the New Year's Honours List for services to horse racing, adding to the MBE he received in 2003 and the OBE in 2010.

And on top of all that, he's a really nice guy who is very pleasant to talk to and is thoroughly good company. I am aware that earlier I said I thought John Francome was the best jockey of them all, and I still stand by that, but there is no arguing that AP was the most successful. I doubt if anyone will get near to his records for a very, very long time.

Aidan O'Brien

The current master of Ballydoyle, Aidan O'Brien is, in my opinion, without question the greatest trainer of horses in racing today. He took over the stables from Vincent O'Brien and you may think, "Ah well, it was obviously in his blood." But he is no relation to the old master and all of Aidan's skills and talents are due to him alone. Well, him and what I believe was the influence of Jim Bolger.

Aidan O'Brien was one of six children and his father was a farmer and small-scale horse trainer in County Wexford, Ireland. Starting his professional working life with P.J. Finn's racing stables at the Curragh, he moved to join Jim Bolger at Coolcullen. Jim's been rightly credited with mentoring and bringing on a number of good jockeys, including as I've mentioned AP McCoy. I don't doubt he fostered the same winning mentality and drive into the young O'Brien.

Aidan took over his wife's training license, who herself was a superb jumps trainer, in 1993 before taking over from the retiring Vincent in Ballydoyle in 1996. Although things didn't go brilliantly straight away, from 2003 there has been a continuous stream of winners that is simply stupendous.

Not quite able to emulate Vincent in the successes spread across the whole of National Hunt and flat, Aidan has tried his best and to date has accumulated on the flat, 29 English Classis wins, 39 Irish Classics, two French Arcs and the Cox Plate in Australia. In National Hunt he won three Champion Hurdles with the legendary Istabraq.

It is true that he's blessed with the pick of the Coolmore stud and has, in Ryan Moore, a phenomenal jockey, but I think his winning mentality and non-stop drive comes from the time he spent under Jim Bolger in County Kilkenny.

When I said Aidan wasn't related to Vincent, that is true, but it seems he is establishing his own 'bloodline'. His son, Joseph who initially started out as a jockey for his father and notched up wins on the flat including a 2,000 Guineas, a St Leger and two Derby victories, has now become a trainer himself.

Starting out in 2016, it would appear that he is definitely a chip off the old block having, in his first full year, taken out Australia's biggest race, the Melbourne Cup, with Rekindling pipping Johannes Vermeer, trained by Aidan, into second. The future, it would seem, is bright at Ballydoyle.

Ryan Moore

Ryan Moore, born in Brighton in 1983, is currently the first choice jockey for Aidan O'Brien's Ballydoyle operation. He also occasionally rides horses for Juddmonte, owned by Prince Khalid bin Abdullah and has been the Queen's jockey, under Sir Michael Stoute, famously winning the Royal Ascot Gold Cup on Estimate for Her Majesty in 2013.

I think he is presently the best jockey in the world and not just thanks to the standard of rides he gets through Aidan. He does, in simple terms, know where the winning post is. Being aware of how he is travelling in a race means he can produce the horse at the right time. That sort of ability is rare.

I was lucky that I was able to start riding early and Ryan was the same, starting out at age four by being a member of the Pony Club. As time went on he didn't want to be a show jumper, instead he fancied National Hunt. AP McCoy rode for Moore's father when in his teens and Ryan, aged twelve, schooled horses with him. He's been quoted as saying he was influenced by AP's drive and dedication. Ryan's first win came when he was only sixteen and that's when he decided to take up racing as a career, but as a flat jockey. He started by riding his grandfather's horses but moved to join Richard Hannon, under whose tutelage he became Champion Apprentice.

As time went on he rode more and more for Sir Michael Stoute and in 2006 won the first of his three flat racing Champion Jockey titles. An ever increasing relationship with Aidan O'Brien at Ballydoyle finally led to him being named as that stable's main jockey from 2015. By the end of the 2017 season, Ryan had over

2,000 winners in Britain alone, making him the third most prolific of all active flat jockeys, behind Frankie Dettori and Joe Fanning, both of whom had been riding for more than ten years longer. He's also got ten English Classics already including two Derby wins.

With all of his success it was interesting to hear him say that he'd never heard a reaction on a racecourse like the one he got winning the Gold Cup at Royal Ascot on the Queen's filly, Estimate. Her Majesty had been there to present the cup to the winning owner, but instead Prince Andrew had to present it to his mother.

Joe Mercer

When I was starting out, Joe Mercer OBE was the man all the young jockeys were told to look to, even though he rode on the flat.

Apart from having been a Champion Apprentice twice over, he won the first of his eight Classic victories, the Oaks, still as an apprentice, which is frankly amazing. Added to that early promise, Joe had style. Real style on the back of a horse.

If you want to teach someone how to ride a horse at speed, then go and get tapes, or YouTube nowadays I suppose, of Joe Mercer riding Brigadier Gerard or Kris or any of his other 2,810 winners stretching over a nearly forty-year riding career.

Mind you, he nearly didn't have half the career when in 1972 he was involved in a plane crash. Thankfully he walked away from it but the pilot, a friend of his, sadly died.

During his spell at Henry Cecil's yard he won his only British flat racing Champion Jockey's title in 1979, but he will always be best remembered for his partnership with Brigadier Gerard, winner of seventeen of his eighteen races between 1970 and 1972. Most notable of these, the 2,000 Guineas in 1971 where he had to beat the later Arc and Derby winner Mill Reef and the amazing French colt My Swallow. It's the calibre of the horses he beat that prompted Joe to say that even Frankel, whilst as good as the Brigadier, wasn't better.

I always thought Joe was the most articulate of jockeys and thought he would have made a great television pundit, but instead, when Smokin' Joe retired as a jockey in 1985, he worked initially as a jockey's agent before accepting a job as racing manager for Maktoum bin Rashid Al Maktoum in 1987. He finally retired from that in 2006.

ANNEX

John Gosden

John Gosden OBE is, in my opinion one of the geniuses of this racing game. As a trainer he has trained over 3,000 winners worldwide, including the big races such as, the Breeders' Cup, the Derby, the Arc, the King George and the Eclipse. To train and win in Europe to that level is difficult, to have over 600 winners in the States as well is almost unbelievable.

John's father was a clever trainer who had also gone to the US and enjoyed a lot of success. John, unlike so many of us, stayed on at school and got an Economics degree from Cambridge. Then he was an assistant trainer to Vincent O'Brien and later, Noel Murless. If you wanted to choose two trainers to learn from it's doubtful you could pick better. After a while he went out to the States and in the early 80's began to make his mark. By the end of that decade he was firmly established as a top US trainer and then he came home to Newmarket. If anyone thought he'd have to wait a while for success in Europe, they were wrong. Within the first two years he trained the winners of the Prix de l'Abbaye de Longchamp, the Irish St. Leger, the Grosser Preis von Baden and Gran Premio di Milano, the Prix de la Forêt and more than 100 other races.

In 1996 he won his first English Classic, the St. Leger and then he added the Derby, with Benny the Dip in 1997. To date he's trained nine Classic winners.

I like John and I know that most of the people I still know in racing agree that he is one of the finest racehorse trainers of his generation. Completely trustworthy, always open and honest I've noticed the strangest thing. If I am in or around a racecourse and an interview with John comes on the TV monitors, everyone stops to listen. I think that says it all.

ANNEX

Frankie Dettori

What can I say that hasn't already been said about the 'Face of Flat Racing'? Frankie Dettori MBE is a force of nature and a brilliant jockey.

The epitome of a fun-loving, cheeky, humorous and engaging man, he combines that with all of his natural Italian effervescence and it's easy to see why, when he walks into a room the attention spotlight falls on him with ease. People however sometimes forget just what an amazing jockey he is.

Famous for his trademark dismounts, he is of course the man who won the entire card, all seven races, on British Champions' Day at Ascot in 1996.

Born Lanfranco Dettori in Milan, Italy in 1970, he came to Britain to be apprentice to trainer Luca Cumani in Newmarket at just fourteen years of age.

In 1990, still only nineteen, he became the first teenager since Lester Piggott to ride 100 winners in one season. Interestingly, he suffered all the same hardships I used to in trying to keep the weight in check and I remember him saying in an interview that, before the Jockey Club bans came into force, he had used 'Piss Pills', diuretics and laxatives, just as I had done.

He lives quite close by in Newmarket and I do see him out and about regularly. Like Joe Mercer, he's the survivor of a light plane crash. Frankie and Ray Cochrane were aboard a Piper Seneca when it crashed on take-off from Newmarket on its way to Goodwood in 2000. Ray Cochrane was awarded the Queen's Commendation for Bravery for helping Frankie away from the aircraft and then trying desperately, but unsuccessfully, to get the pilot out.

After recovering from that ordeal, Frankie returned to racing. To describe him as a rider, well you can only say, he is simply world class. He does all of the aspects of riding so well and his seventeen English Classic victories added to his record-breaking five Prix de l'Arc de Triomphe wins are testimony to how hard he works. Still riding at the top levels of the game at age forty-six is also proof of how remarkable his fitness regime is. The strength and the simple 'puff' or wind you need as a jockey is not that well understood, and indeed was one of my main concerns when I was trying to come back from the chemo treatment, so to maintain it into your forties is no mean feat.

I think for me, Frankie is also a fantastic example of the internationalism that is modern day racing. In his career he has scored major victories in significant races in twenty-two other nations besides Britain. Obviously some of the countries you would guess, like Ireland, the US and France, but add in the A J Moir Stakes in Australia, three Dubai World Cups in the UAE plus Hong Kong, Singapore, Italy (of course) and some more unusual venues like Trinidad and Tobago, Bahrain and Switzerland to name but a few. Everywhere he goes he is recognised and I wonder if he isn't the first true international superstar of racing? Whether he is or not, he has been a great ambassador for our sport and when the likes of Lester Piggott says he is the best jockey riding today, who can argue?

Lester Piggot

I think the legend and genius of the 'Long Fellow', Lester Piggott, will never be surpassed. In my opinion, he is the best flat jockey there ever was. I was in awe of him when I was a boy and still am to be honest. I know many will say it was Sir Gordon Richards (who is the last profile in this book) and he certainly had more winners, but I still think Lester had the edge, mainly due to the calibre of the races he won. Thirty Classic victories including nine Derby wins was unprecedented and I doubt will ever be beaten.

Unlike some jockeys and trainers I've talked about in here, who had no or little family background in horse racing, Lester could trace his pedigree back like a thoroughbred race horse.

His grandfather Ernie Piggott rode three Grand National winners, in 1912, 1918 and 1919 and was married to a sister of two jockeys who both rode Derby winners. Ernie was also three-times National Hunt Champion Jockey. On retiring from riding, he had a stables in Letcombe Regis.

Lester's father, Keith was also a successful National Hunt jockey, winning the Champion Hurdle in 1939. He established a trainer's yard in Lambourn after he stopped riding and trained a Grand National winner, Ayala in 1963. He went on to lift the Champion Trainer title in the 62/63 season.

With that sort of bloodline you'd have thought Lester would have been a jump jockey, but as a young man he went onto the flat and to say he caused a sensation is an understatement. He rode his first Epsom Derby winner, on Never Say Die, in 1954 at the tender age of eighteen. He also caused a stir with his vastly different and revolutionary riding style, which ended up being copied by the majority of jockeys.

Being 5ft 8inches he was very tall for a jockey and the struggles he had with his weight make mine look like child's play. Throughout his career he would consistently get down to not much more than 8st. That meant he was about twenty-five to thirty full pounds under his normal weight levels. As a mark of the man's dedication to his profession I don't think you can get a clearer example.

Champion Jockey eleven times, he was renowned as having a competitive streak and yet he is such a quiet and unassuming man when you meet him. The thing I find possibly the most remarkable is that the thirtieth of his Classic victories came in the 2,000 Guineas in 1992 on board Rodrigo de Triano. Lester was fifty-five years old.

To ride for leisure at fifty-five is trying. To ride professionally is hard. To win a Classic? Well, I just don't know how you do that.

Henry Cecil

Henry, or Sir Henry Richard Amherst Cecil as he was to be after getting his deserved knighthood in 2011, was a brilliant, ten times Champion Trainer. He just seemed to understand horses and I don't think there was ever a better trainer of a mare or a filly in racing.

I honestly remember watching him one day and wondering, 'God, can he actually hear what that horse is thinking?' It just looked like he had that knack. Funnily enough, my inkling about his training style was confirmed by the man himself when he was interviewed once and said, "I do everything by instinct really, not by the book. I like to think I've got a feeling for and understand my horses, that they tell me what to do really."

Henry was born in Aberdeenshire in 1943, and his father had been in the Parachute Regiment. Sadly he didn't make it home from the war and his mother remarried later to Captain Cecil Boyd-Rochfort, who was British flat racing's Champion Trainer five times and who trained for, among others, George VI.

Henry had an early period of remarkable success from the 1960's through to the 1990s when he won everything set before him. In 1999 he surpassed himself by winning the 1,000 Guineas, the Oaks and the Derby and finishing second in the 2,000 Guineas and the St Leger. It was a brilliant demonstration of the trainer's knack in getting his horses ready at the right time. But then, it all went downhill and fast. A lot of his owners retired and some, for various reasons, moved their horses, including forty owned by Maktoum bin Rashid Al Maktoum.

It looked like Henry should call it a day, and between July 2000 and October 2006, he failed to train a winner in any Group

One race, but he persisted and thank goodness he did. His later successes, beginning when he won the Oaks in 2007, saw the coming of a legend.

I believe that only Henry Cecil could have brought on Prince Khaled Abdulla's horse, Frankel in the manner that allowed him to excel. Unbeaten in his fourteen-race career, with lifetime earnings of nearly £3M, the highest-rated racehorse in the world since May 2011 and now commanding a stud value of £100M and that's apparently a conservative estimate, I believe it was all due to the genius of the gentleman that was Henry Cecil.

Yes, jockeys surely have their part to play, and the natural capacity and potential of the horse has to be in there, but to bring it out again and again and again requires the consummate training professional. Mind you, given all the horses he ever trained, even Henry himself said of Frankel, "He's the best I've ever had, the best I've ever seen."

Henry was yet another friend of mine who I would lose to cancer. He succumbed to stomach cancer in June 2013 and his passing was quite rightly marked with a minute's silence at Royal Ascot the following week. He was an exceptionally generous and kind man.

Steve Cauthen

I first met Steve Cauthern when I was out in the States riding for Burly and Jonathan. He was 'The Kid' back then and at seventeen, in only his second year of riding, he became the first jockey to win $6M in a single season. Like I said, the US knew how to pay prize money.

The following year he earned even more and in 1978, became the youngest jockey to ever win the US Triple Crown. In fact, he was the last Triple Crown winning jockey until 2015. Proof if ever you needed it of how hard some racing triples are to win.

I think he was the best jockey ever to come from America and ride in England. In 1979, struggling to make the very light US riding weights he decided the higher weights in the UK and Europe would be more achievable. On his arrival, he set his stall out early by winning his first ever ride in the UK. Over the next decade and a half he'd go on to win the Champion Jockey championship three times and lift ten English Classics, including the 1,000 and 2,000 Guineas, the Derby twice, three St Legers and three Oaks.

In 1985, not content with the US Triple Crown, he won the English flat racing 'Fillies' Triple Crown' with victories in the 1,000 Guineas, the Oaks and the St. Leger on the Henry Cecil trained, Oh So Sharp. This winning of the Fillie's Triple is an achievement which to date (2017) hasn't since been repeated.

In 1989, he won both the French and Irish Derbies and in 1991 he won the Italian variant. After retiring he returned to the States and bought a stud farm.

Personally, I felt he was second only to Lester Piggott in terms of pure racing ability and was the perfect judge of a race. His situational awareness and ability to know when to press was on a different level and with a career total of 2,794 winners his record speaks for itself.

Peter Easterby

A fellow Yorkshire man, Miles Henry 'Peter' Easterby is the absolute epitome of a self-made man within racing. From humble beginnings in a tiny stables near Malton in 1950, Peter became the most successful dual-purpose trainer in British horseracing history with over 1,000 winners on both flat and National Hunt, a feat equalled by no one.

With a shrewd eye for a potential champion thoroughbred, he once said, "You've got to use your eyes. You only have to look at 'em to know if they're right or wrong," he eventually trained some of the best racing stock in the land and principal amongst them were the two legends, Night Nurse and Sea Pigeon.

The former was the Champion Hurdle winner in 1976 and 1977, a race that was famously described by the Racing Post as the 'strongest field ever assembled' but not content with this amazing hurdles pedigree, Peter trained him for the Cheltenham Gold Cup, only narrowly missing out to yet another Easterby trained runner, Little Owl in 1981. Having just failed to become the first horse to complete the Cheltenham Champion Hurdle-Gold Cup double, Night Nurse would go on to get a Timeform rating of 182, the highest ever awarded to a hurdler.

The latter of those two legends, Sea Pigeon, arguably managed even greater feats. He won the Champion Hurdle in 1980 and 1981 and also won the Ebor Handicap and Chester Cup (x2) in flat racing. His second Hurdles triumph saw him become the oldest horse ever to win it and John Francome's ride on him that day is probably one of the most outstanding efforts you'll ever see in racing. By the time Sea Pigeon was retired in 1982, he was as famous with the general public as Arkle and Red Rum.

Of course these two horses only represent the pinnacle of a vast training career that saw Peter win an outstanding thirteen times at the Cheltenham Festival alone, including two Gold Cups, three Arkle Trophies and the Champion Hurdle five times. This last was a record only just surpassed by Nicky Henderson in 2017. To win five Champion Hurdles is remarkable and many trainers would dream of winning one and be content. Of course Peter didn't just excel at Cheltenham, or indeed just in National Hunt and his flat racing triumphs were just as prodigious.

I must admit, I always liked Peter. He was and still is a plain-speaking, forthright Yorkshire man who knows racing. From that 1950 yard with borrowed numbers of horses just to get his trainer's license, he went on to establish himself as a legend and now, his son Tim seems to be carrying on the family tradition, having already trained a classic winner in the shape of Bollin Eric, who took out the St Leger in 2002. To solidify the Easterby legacy further, grandson William is an adept amateur flat and jump jockey.

I do wonder if anyone will ever equal or surpass the 1,000 winners on both flat and jumps, but if they do, they'll have had to be the equal to a genius.

Gordon Richards

Last, but by no means least, in my selected look at jockeys and trainers is the man who without question has the most Jockey Championships and winners to his name.

Sir Gordon Richards was born in 1904, the son of a coal miner and grew up in Shropshire. He started riding his father's pit ponies at a very young age and by only seven he was driving a pony and trap in the family business.

A stable boy at 15, to Jimmy White it wasn't long before his natural talent was evident. He won his first race at Leicester in 1921 at just 17 years of age.

He came out of his apprenticeship in 1925 and made a good start to his career by winning the Champion Jockey title in his first season with a total of 118 wins, a remarkable number that he more than doubled in 1932 to 259 wins. That record stood until 1947, when he broke it again with a phenomenal 269 winners.

It says something that it took AP McCoy until 2002 to surpass that number of winners in a season and he had a lot more rides in which to do it than Gordon did. Even then, Gordon's total of 4,870 winners in his career is still at the top of the list. I can't ever see anyone beating it.

However this could have been a very different story as he was struck down with tuberculosis in 1926 and recuperated from his illness in a Norfolk sanctuary, which meant he had to stop riding. It's a testament to how good he was that he was back in the saddle by December 1926 and returned to winning ways in the 1927 season.

Despite all of these winners though, for the majority of his career, the biggest prize in flat racing, the Epsom Derby eluded him. I remember growing up with all the stories and even recall being told about how Gordon had won four of the five classics in a single season, 1942, but still couldn't win a Derby. In fact it would take him until 1953, when he was forty-nine years old, to achieve the biggest win of his career. In front of the Queen, in what was her Coronation year, he won on Pinza, who at 16-hands was a huge horse for a Derby runner. I've seen old Pathé newsreel footage of the race and the roar that greeted his sweeping run up the final furlongs was huge.

Ironic that this most popular of wins came at the cost of beating the newly crowned Queen's horse into second. It would have been quite the Coronation year if she'd won a Derby as well, but she obviously bore no ill will as before the year was out she had conferred on Gordon a knighthood. As yet the only one ever to be given to a flat jockey.

Due to an injury Sir Gordon retired from riding in 1954, but first as a trainer and then after 1970 as a Racing Manager, he maintained his contact with the sport. I had the great pleasure of meeting him on a number of occasions before his death in 1986 and he was as you would imagine for a man of his generation. Charming, polite and above all, humble. A true gentleman who inspired the love of the nation and who brought the majesty and beauty of horse racing to the masses.

Index

Bob Champion Cancer Trust

We work to help raise money for male cancer research. If you'd like us to attend your event, are thinking of fundraising or would simply like to offer a donation, you can find out more here:

www.bobchampion.org.uk

Telephone: 00 44 (0) 20-7924 3553

Email: info@bobchampion.org.uk

If you have a story to share, we'd love to hear from you.

Injured Jockeys Fund

The Injured Jockeys Fund provides much needed support to those jockeys past or present who are injured, unable to ride, or generally in need. They helped me and thousands of others just like me.

If you can help or would like to know more:

Telephone: 00 44 (0) 1638 662246

www.injuredjockeys.co.uk

We'd like to say a special thank you to the following people, without who's help and kindness this book would certainly not have had as many images!

The Liverpool Echo
Jean-Pierre Montbazet
Julie Voules
Simon Massen
Margaret Neesham
Charles Betz
The Bob Champion Cancer Trust

FCM Publishing

For Creative Minds

I sincerely hope you enjoyed this book.

If you'd like to know more about our forthcoming titles, authors and special events, or to be notified of early releases then email us at:

follow@fcmmedia.co.uk or come find us on the web at:

www.fcmpublishing.co.uk or on Twitter at:

@fcmtaryn

We love what we do and we'd like you to be part of a thriving community of people who enjoy books and the very best reading experiences.

Taryn Johnston
Creative Director
FCM Media Group

Lightning Source UK Ltd.
Milton Keynes UK
UKHW010630161218
333983UK00010B/1218/P